To my good friends
Tammy & George
Love
Larry Lamb

The Weighting Game

The Truth About Weight Control

by Lawrence E. Lamb, M.D.

Lyle Stuart Inc.   Secaucus, New Jersey

Published by Lyle Stuart, Inc.
120 Enterprise Ave., Secaucus, N.J. 07094
Published simultaneously in Canada by
Musson Book Company,
A division of General Publishing Co. Limited
Don Mills, Ontario

Address queries regarding rights and permissions
to Lyle Stuart, Inc., 120 Enterprise Ave.,
Secaucus, N.J. 07094

Manufactured in the United States of America

ISBN 0-8184-0487-6

Foreword

Do you think you need to lose weight? Are you limiting your calories to avoid gaining weight? If so, you are probably vulnerable to misguided and often harmful advice. If you are overweight, you know what discrimination is. Our society discriminates against people who are overweight. It is often believed these people are underexercised and overfed. This may be the case, but the belief that this is all there is to being overweight is a dangerous oversimplification. Many "overweight" people are perfectly normal and have simply inherited the genes that make them what they are, just as people inherit genes to be black, white or some shade in between. It is just as wrong to discriminate against "overweight" people as it is to discriminate against a person because of his race or religion. This prejudicial attitude in our culture has caused many normal people to have a poor self image, and many others to be victims of a long list of scams dependent on misconceptions about weight control.

The widely held mistaken beliefs about weight control have made it possible to take advantage of people who are either overweight or think they are. One of the best examples is the plethora of diet books that don't work or are even dangerous for the public. The complete failure of this approach to weight control is evidenced by the fact that well over 90 percent of the people who lose weight by such popular diets regain what they lost.

Despite the fact that for over 25 years the nation's best authorities on nutrition and metabolism have pointed out the misrepresentations, mistakes and unsound advice in many of these books, publishers continue to promote them. I have been told by some editors of some publishing companies that they want a "hook" to stimulate impulse buying. In other words, they are not really interested in helping people with weight control, but in making money off the person who thinks he or she needs to lose weight. From there, you can go on to the extravagant misleading or false claims you see advertised in the papers. The overweight person, or the person who thinks he or she is overweight, is their victim. The individuals who promote weight loss hoaxes are no different from the quacks who promote phony cures for cancer and arthritis.

I decided to write this book because the public badly needs to know how body weight is controlled rather than more vague diet advice. I know how badly this information is needed from the thousands of letters I receive each year as a result of my syndicated health column. There are millions of people who are on diets that cause significant health problems. As a cardiologist who helped to launch many of the programs to help prevent heart disease, I am an enthusiastic supporter of using a low-fat, low-cholesterol diet to help prevent heart attacks and strokes. As a physician involved in providing useful information to the general public, I am equally aware of the problems of undernutrition that have been caused by misrepresenting the truth about the factors that control body weight.

I believe undernutrition is now a national problem in the adult population of the United States. It is responsible for millions of people having lost their zest for living.

Another matter that has increasingly concerned me is the preoccupation with how many calories a person consumes. That seems to be all diet books talk about. The problem of being overweight depends on both the calories consumed and the calories used. There has been shockingly little attention given to how the body eliminates calories. Most people have no idea that most of the calories they consume are eliminated as heat—much less that this is done through the skin. Put another way, calories go in through your mouth and come out through your skin.

The public, and many professionals, do not understand the importance of developing large, strong muscles in helping to prevent being overweight. Many think jogging or running is the answer—but it is only part of the answer.

Too much of the approach of weight reduction is based on one idea:

"You eat too much." A look at all the aspects that determine whether or not you are overweight is long overdue. People need to know more about what controls their body weight than just the calories in their diets. When people understand the role of the brain, genes, exercise, and loss of calories through the skin, as well as their diet, they can begin to make informed choices regarding what they should or should not do about their weight. They will know how to use a diet properly for weight control. When the public understands what controls body weight, hopefully many prejudices will be stamped out.

I hope this book will cause a renewed interest among professionals in measuring, on an individual basis, what each person's real calorie requirements are, rather than taking the short cut of factory-made diets and standard weight tables for everyone. It would be nice to see people studied to find out how much oxygen they require, so their individual calorie needs could be assessed more accurately.

Gaining an understanding of what controls body weight is the best protection people can have against being ripped-off by unsound diet books, diet pills, body wraps, sweat suits, passive exercise machines, unwise surgery and various fads that promise quick weight loss without pain. It is essential to protect people from weight loss programs that are damaging to their health. I hope this book, which tells the reader the truth about weight control, will help the public with this important health problem.

If a look at the total picture of weight control in this book helps to bring new reason to the weighting game, I will be satisfied.

LAWRENCE E. LAMB, M.D.

Contents

Chapter 1

Yes, There Is a Secret

DEAR DR. LAMB: I am a 32-year-old female, 5 feet 7 and weigh 180 pounds. My friend, who was the same weight, also female, and I started an exercise and diet program three months ago. She has lost 20 pounds and is still losing. To my surprise I have not lost a pound.

We both had complete physicals and are in perfect health. We walk three miles twice a week, work out 20 minutes on weights and a sit-up board every day. We eat one meal a day from the basic four food groups, take vitamins and drink plenty of fluids, which include milk, juice and coffee. Our total calorie intake is less than 1,000 calories a day. Our jobs are similar. What is wrong with me? Should I just stop eating entirely and just exercise and drink fluids?

This is just one of the thousands of letters I have received from people trying to lose weight. The story of these two women shows that there is much more to losing pounds of unwanted body fat than just a diet, or even a diet and exercise program. The factors involved in weight control are not at all simple, and are far more complicated than a quickie diet program. It really is true that a person can be on a very restricted diet, follow a vigorous exercise program and not lose weight, just as this woman has described. In many cases it is not true that the reason people don't lose weight is because they are consuming lots of calories. If it were as simple as a diet, most people would not have a problem in shedding unwanted pounds.

There are millions of people counting the calories in their food. Many of them are estimating how many calories they use up with their exercise, whether it is jogging, aerobic dancing or a workout at their favorite health spa. Multimillion dollar industries have sprung up to help people eat low calorie foods and drink low calorie beverages, or to "burn off calories." It's in to be thin. A really healthy person should have well-defined muscles rippling as they contract under his skin without being encased in fat. The irony of all this is that while everyone participating in the weighting game is counting calories in and used with exercise, no one seems to be talking about the real way your body loses calories. A major factor in determining whether you are fat or not is how your body eliminates calories. You lose calories through your skin, and how your skin does that is controlled by your brain. This woman who cannot lose weight was probably not designed to weigh less than she does. It may be unhealthy for her to lose body fat, and her brain sets in motion the body's mechanisms to keep her from losing weight. *Not everyone was designed to be thin.* Millions of people who cannot accept themselves as they are, create psychological problems for themselves by trying to be thinner than they are meant to be. The best example is the young woman with anorexia nervosa who actually starves herself in an attempt to be thin.

Being overweight can be unhealthy. It is important that many people today have learned this lesson, and have adopted more healthy lifestyles. But it is equally important for you to know that you can also be too thin. It is not just the young girl suffering from a false body image who may damage her health with unwise dietary habits. Millions of adults are suffering from undernutrition and do not know it. Are you a victim of undernutrition? I don't mean a vitamin deficiency, although that can be a problem too, but a calorie deficiency. Are you tired all the time and have to force yourself to do anything physical? That is common in people who do not consume enough calories. Fatigue makes it more difficult to push yourself to be physically active. If you are inactive, that does limit how effective your body is at eliminating calories. In many people a vicious cycle develops. When they don't eat enough because they want to lose weight, they decrease their physical activity, use fewer calories, and can't lose weight. More and more stringent calorie restriction is not the answer.

Are you on a low calorie diet but can't lose weight? Millions are. At one time doctors thought all these people were cheating on their diets. Many of them are not. They are telling the truth when they claim they are consuming fewer than 1,000 calories a day and haven't lost a pound. The secret in many of these cases is to increase the ways the body loses calories. Many others, who can't lose weight, should not be trying to lose more body fat. Their bodies have shut down their calorie losing mechanisms in order to protect their health.

A surprising fact is that increasing the calorie intake actually may not cause you to gain weight. You can find out how many calories your body needs when you are not active by simply having the amount of oxygen your body uses measured. It is based on an old principle that seems largely forgotten in the heyday of counting calories and fad diets. Small individuals may not require a lot of calories. If your calorie requirement is indeed very low, there may be a medical reason for it, or it may be related to your lifestyle.

There are secrets to exercising, too. Many unfortunate individuals do limit their calorie intake and exercise a reasonable amount. Still they do not lose weight, even though there is nothing wrong with them medically. Again, the body may be sending them a message that they don't need to lose weight. Also, it may relate to how they exercise. Not all exercise is equal in terms of stimulating your body to lose calories. The explanation for that fact is in the different ways exercise causes your body to lose calories.

I will give you a sound concept on how to influence your body's function as a calorie exchanger, but it is important for you to realize that pushing these methods to the extreme may not be wise. We are all individuals. While some people really need to lose pounds of body fat, others do not. You may be one of those who does not need to lose weight.

I'm sure you have seen some people who seem to be able to eat unlimited amounts of food, are not especially active and still don't gain a pound, while the next person seems to be able to walk through the dining room and gain weight. Yes, this really happens. Yes, there is a secret why one person loses and the other one does not. The secret is locked within the brain. I do not mean you can just wish to lose weight and have it disappear by magic, and I don't mean you can do it with "will power." There is more to it than rigidly controlling the number of calories you consume.

One of the sad truths of the weighting game is that more than 90 percent of people who lose weight gain it back. For many, it's 10 pounds off and 15 pounds on. What else can you expect when people return to the same habits they had before they started on a diet? But many of these people really do not return to the same lifestyle they had before, and still they regain their weight. How is this possible? It's simple. Your body is very efficient, and it stops eliminating calories that your brain thinks you need. It may take a while, but eventually your brain will win. There is another problem involved. Many people following fad diets actually lose muscle and other body cells. These cells are very important to how your body processes calories. When you lose these, your body is apt to need fewer calories than it did before you began to diet. With a decrease in daily requirements for calories, you gradually regain the calories you lost.

Often it is healthy to go on a diet and exercise program, which does eliminate calories, even though a person may still weigh the same, or even gain weight. People find this frustrating, but they really should be pleased, because it means improved health, whereas weight loss alone may be harmful. How can you lose calories and not lose weight, or actually gain weight? If you develop good healthy muscles, at the time you are eliminating body fat, you can actually be losing calories and gaining weight. If you need to lose body fat, you should really be losing calories, not necessarily pounds of body weight. The two are not the same.

People do tend to gain weight when they reach middle age. This is such a common event that it is called the middle-aged spread. It doesn't happen to everyone, but it is the norm. This seems to be more common in women, and they are often very distressed by this change in their appearance. Many of them interpret the middle-aged spread as meaning they are no longer young and beautiful. In a society that places a premium on youth, that is often hard to accept. In the quest to be "forever young," many go on crash diets and exercise programs to defeat the process. It is reasonable to question whether it really is wise to try to fool Mother Nature.

In recent decades there has been a growing misconception of what a woman should look like. Fashion models have set goals that are not realistic, or healthy, for most women. When a person cannot lose weight, he or she often develops a guilt complex. This undermines a person's ego. When anyone thinks his or her appearance is bad, this then causes a poor self-image. The thought is reinforced by other people's reactions. Often, a person is in a weight control program, and the program supervisor adds to the problem by refusing to accept that the dieter has not gone off the diet and eaten forbidden food. In other cases, the appetite stimulation has won out, and the person has indeed given in to an overwhelming desire for food. Actually, the forces of nature have won, but the victim doesn't view the situation that way and has a real guilt trip.

The truth is that a certain amount of body fat in the right places is part of being female. The change begins at puberty. Before sex hormones start changing a little girl's body, she may not have a lot of body fat and may be more muscular. Both males and females look a lot alike until hormones work their magic. The release of the sex hormones that cause these changes at this stage of life is controlled by the brain. Female hormones cause the development of fat deposits over the buttocks and in the breast. These increased fat deposits are responsible for the shape of the female torso. They are part of a girl's secondary sexual characteristics. A girl who retains her androgynous characteristics has failed to develop her secondary sexual characteristics, and biologically is not as feminine as the girl who has undergone the normal changes. It is normal for females to have more body fat than males. When little boys start developing muscles, little girls start developing fat deposits in the right places to help them fulfill their future biological roles as mothers. The young girl who fails to develop normal fat deposits may also be laying the groundwork for future medical problems.

A girl's development of body fat at puberty is a good example of how your body has a script that determines how much fat you should have and where it should be at different stages of your life. It is as regular as the other changes that are part of your biological script. Your baby teeth erupt on schedule and are lost on schedule. Permanent teeth also follow a program. Your long bones fuse at a specific time, signaling the end of growth in height. The menopause occurs on schedule in most women and body fat stores that affect a person's appearance are no different. Your body will work hard to help you fulfill the script you were born with, whether you like that script or not. A failure to recognize this has led to prejudicial attitudes toward people who were born to carry more body fat than others. This attitude of society reinforces a person's feeling of guilt about being overweight and is a powerful driving force to try still one more unhealthy diet to lose weight.

When many women reach middle age, often they are again programmed to develop more body fat. That body fat plays a role in keeping them feminine. You may be surprised to know that body fat is important to a woman's hormone level. Although her ovaries may not be producing the same amount of estrogen as they did during the child-bearing years, they are still producing sex hormones. One of these, androstenedione, is acted on by body fat cells to produce estrone, an estrogen. That extra estrogen helps to protect a woman from the problems of estrogen deficiency, including bone loss that causes osteoporosis. It is not surprising that a woman's body fights her efforts to look like a teen-ager. It is not wise to fight your body. Those fad diets that many use at that stage of life can wreck their health.

Does that mean your body needs some fat? Of course it does. Fat is the calorie reserve that we still have to help us survive a period of starvation. Modern man, in our developed countries, is not usually faced with such a survival situation, but many people in the world still have to face that problem. Even in our overfed society, a person may have a medical disorder that will either require more calories than he will get, or one that will keep him from eating normally. A healthy amount of fat stores may see him through an emergency. Fat also is useful in helping your body resist cold, and it cushions your body. The fat inside your abdomen provides support for your abdominal organs. Without this normal support, the abdominal organs tend to fall to the bottom of your abdominal cavity, a condition called visceroptosis. While it is not healthy to be too thin, there are middle-aged individuals who do need to lose excess body fat for health reasons. We are all individuals, no one rule applies to all. Before you decide to lose a lot of weight, you need to know whether it would be healthy for you. Even if you want to do it for the sake of your appearance, it is wise to consider the health implications.

Other than the question of whether your skin is going to be wrinkled or have stretch marks, you may never have thought of your skin as a factor in being overweight. Almost all the calories that are eliminated from your body are eliminated as heat. You may not have realized that a calorie is a unit of heat. The basic studies that underlie what your body does with food were based on the heat energy (calories) in food, and how the body eliminated these calories of heat. You can actually measure this heat energy directly.

The truth is, we all have a hot body. If you want to warm up a room, all you have to do is put a lot of people in it. When you are at rest, all of the calories eliminated from your body are eliminated through your skin. Your skin is your cooling system. If you had no way to eliminate the calories of heat released by your body's metabolism of foods, your body temperature would soar. In fact, that is exactly how you develop a fever. Your brain simply shuts down the heat-loss mechanism and the body temperature rises.

Your brain and the nerves connected to it control the blood flow through your skin, which is of major importance in eliminating calories. It also controls the sweat glands. Sweating is an important mechanism in losing calories through your skin. Thus, not only does your brain control the calories you consume, but it also controls how calories are eliminated from your body. Evidently, it also does one other thing. On the basis of your life script it determines, within a given range, how much body fat you should have at different stages of your life, as occurs with the changes at puberty and at middle life. You can override these actions, but the optimal level for your body fat is evidently set by a script carried out by your brain. It not only controls how much fat, but also where it should go.

Though the brain controls how many calories you ingest, it can be influenced. Certain medical problems that are associated with obesity actually cause the brain to stimulate a person to increase his calorie intake. This also happens with some forms of brain damage. Psychological factors can cause a person to overeat. But again this is accomplished through the brain. The brain really is the central control for how many calories you consume, and what happens to them. No wonder it is the most important organ in determining whether a person is overweight or not.

You may have thought that whether you are fat or not depends upon your endocrine glands. They are quite important, but these glands are largely controlled by your brain. The brain has its own rhythms that control the secretion of hormones from the endocrine glands. The rhythm for a woman's menstrual cycle is determined by her brain. Your brain releases chemicals that tell your pituitary gland, located under your brain, when to signal the sex glands to release hormones. The natural rhythm for males and females is different. Your thyroid gland is also influenced by your brain.

Does exercise have any role in this? Of course. Exercise may be the best and most healthy way to avoid being overweight. It isn't just the mechanical energy used in exercise that helps. Exercise actually causes the brain to turn on your heat-loss mechanism to help your body to eliminate calories, and it does so by stimulating the loss of calories of heat through your skin.

Do you feel hot or cold? That may be an indicator of whether you really need to lose fat or not. People feel hot when a lot of hot blood circulates through the skin. They feel cold when the blood flow through the skin is diminished. If you really are hot and fat, you are probably consuming more calories than you should.

By now you may be wondering if I am going to tell you that calories don't count. Forget it. *Calories do count.* Those repeated statements by qualified nutritionists about calorie intake controlling body fat are absolutely true. But the secret is, there is more to being fat or thin than the amount of calories you consume, or the number you use in physical activity. Your body is very clever at controlling what happens to the calories you consume. The basic laws of nature don't change, only the way your body responds. The number of calories you ingest will equal the amount of calories your body uses, plus the number of calories stored as fat, but you can significantly influence how many calories your body uses.

As I explain how your body really processes calories in the weighting game, I will add important related factors, but for now I would like for you to think of your body as a simple old-fashioned wood stove. When you put wood in the stove and it is burned with oxygen, the wood releases calories of heat. These calories pass out of the stove through its sides to warm the room. In its simplest concept, your body handles calories the same way. You consume calories as food. The food is oxidized to release calories, and those calories escape your body through your skin. Of course your body is more complicated. Your brain controls the energy you put into your body, and it controls the way the calories escape.

Because of its controls, the body is much like a modern room with air conditioning and central heating. Think of your body as a large room. At one end of the room is a furnace that uses fuel to produce calories of heat to warm the room. At the other end of the room is an air conditioner to eliminate calories of heat. There is a little black control box at the top of the room. It is connected to a thermostat. When the room temperature drops, the thermostat senses that, and through the little black box turns on the furnace to raise the temperature in the room. If the room gets too hot, the thermostat senses that, too. It relays a signal to the little black box. The little black box relays

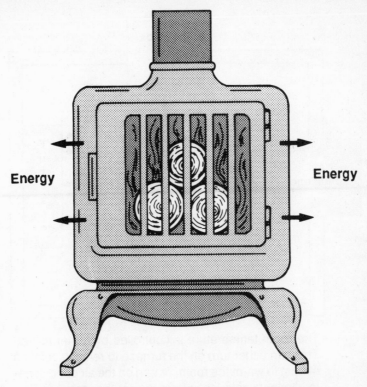

Wood burned in a stove releases energy through the
sides of the stove.

the signal to turn on the air conditioner, which runs until the room
temperature is at the desired level.

Now that is a very simple concept, but it is actually how your body
works. That little black box is your brain, and it does contain a thermostat. The heater is your metabolic furnace that burns food to release
energy. Your cells do this. The air conditioner is your skin, and it
eliminates heat. That is the basic model, and its operation determines
whether you are fat or thin. The way cells release heat by using oxygen is rather well known. How the body eliminates heat is also well
known. But some things are not yet known. What is in the little black
box and how does it work? It will be years before all the questions are
answered, but you don't need to know the specifics of how the black

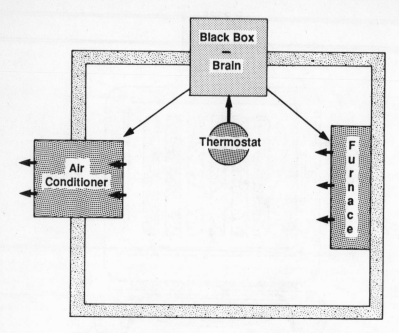

The room temperature is controlled by a thermostat.
This can either turn on the furnace to release calories
of heat to warm the room, or turn on the air conditioner
to eliminate calories of heat to cool the room.

box is wired to know how it affects your body, any more than you need
to know how your automobile works to burn fuel to drive down the
block. It is important that you know that the brain controls it, and it is
equally important for you to have a concept of how your body eliminates calories. Otherwise you will be another victim of the weighting
game, going from one crash diet program to another, perhaps harming
your health and never really being successful.

There is one other large group of people vitally concerned about the
weighting game. I get letters from such individuals all the time. These
are the people who want to gain weight. A young man writes,

DEAR DR. LAMB: I eat like a horse and never gain an ounce. I'm
21 years old, 5 feet 8 inches tall and weigh 128 pounds. I've weighed
this much as long as I can remember. I don't understand it because I'm

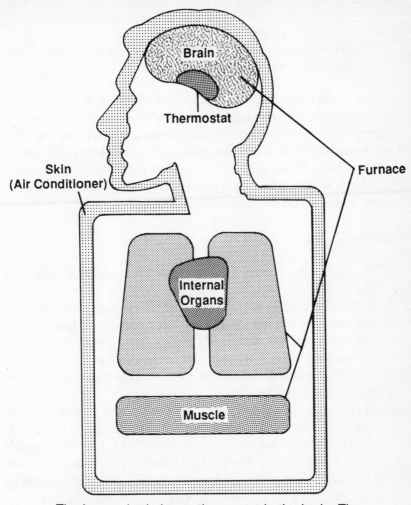

The human body has a thermostat in the brain. The brain controls the air-conditioning mechanism of the skin to cool the body and eliminate calories of heat released inside the body.

always the last one to leave the table. Some people tell me I have a tapeworm.

I don't work. I ride my bicycle every now and then. When I was 14 I started pumping weights. All that did was give me muscle tone. You would not believe the muscle tone I have. My muscles are defined to the max. I still work out with weights now and then, but it has no effect. My muscles don't get bigger, only tighter.

When I eat I stop because I get tired of the taste, or my jaw gets tired from eating. What needs to be done?

Many of the letters are from young men who want to "beef up." Others are from women who want a little more shape. The basic concepts of how your body processes calories apply to them as well. Their brain, and how it controls calories in and calories out, controls their body fat as well. The weighting game really applies to everyone. It is important to everyone to play it right, in order to be a healthy, energetic person, and not a victim.

Summary

1. The factors that control your body weight are controlled by your brain.
2. Your brain controls your appetite and the calories consumed.
3. You lose most of your calories through your skin as heat.
4. Your brain controls the loss of calories through your skin by controlling circulation to the skin and your sweating.
5. Over 90 pecent of all people who lose weight on various programs regain the weight they lost.
6. You have an optimal weight for different stages of your life, and your body makes many adjustments to try to maintain that proper weight for you. That is why it is especially hard for some people to lose weight and equally hard for others to gain weight. It is also why body weight usually tends to remain rather stable despite wide variations in calorie intake and levels of physical activity.

Chapter 2

Your Hot Calories

How many calories are in a piece of bread? In a glass of milk? In a slice of melon? How many calories do you use walking a mile? Everyone in the weighting game talks about calories, but few really know the fascinating story about calories and weight control. Calories are the scientific basis for weight control. Did you know they are really a measure of heat? That's right, when you talk about the number of calories in your favorite food, you are talking about its heat energy. That heat energy is directly related to how much oxygen your body uses, and it is all based on the most fundamental laws of energy, discovered by some of the foremost scientists in the world. The concepts are simple, but essential to playing the weighting game.

What Is a Calorie?

A calorie is the amount of heat energy required to raise 1 milliliter (ml) of water 1 degree Centigrade (C)—from 15 to 16 degrees C. That is a very small unit of energy, but when you talk about calories in your food, or used in activity, you are actually talking about kilocalories. A kilocalorie is 1,000 calories, or the amount of heat required to heat one liter of water (little more than a quart) from 15 to 16 degrees C. In scientific writing, these kilocalories are designated with a capital C, while the small calorie is designated with a small c, but that rule has not been followed consistently and most people just say calories, even though the correct term is kilocalorie. *(To avoid confusion I will use the common term calorie in the remainder of this discussion, although*

I am really talking about kilocalories.) When you walk a mile, you will probably need 60 calories more than you would need if you sat still during that period of time. That glass of protein fortified skim milk probably contains 100 calories.

A calorie is a unit for measuring energy. The weighting game is really about energy. Though we all say the body *uses* energy, it really does not. You can't use up or destroy energy. You can only convert it to other forms of energy. Your body actually *converts* energy. *You literally run on solar energy*. Energy from the sun is trapped by plants and used to combine water and carbon dioxide to form carbohydrates. The very name "carbohydrate" really means a hydrate of carbon. The use of solar energy to form carbohydrates is the beginning of the food chain process that then progresses to form amino acids for protein and fatty acids for fats. When you consume any of these; carbohydrates, proteins, fats or even alcohol, you are filling your metabolic furnace with hydrocarbons.* Yes, our food is made up of hydrocarbons, and like oil, coal and gas is a source for energy. Food heats your body just as other hydrocarbons heat your home or provide the energy to power your automobile. When your body breaks down food hydrocarbons, the process provides the energy you need to run your body.

Think of a flame, whether it is from burning gas, wood, coal or some other energy source. That flame releases energy from whatever is burning. The process is very similar to what happens inside your body. The frequently used phrase "burning off fat" is not as far-fetched as it sounds. Why? Because that flame means oxygen is combining with the hydrocarbon being burned. Chemists call it oxidation. There can be no flame, and no heat energy released, if there is no oxygen available. When the hydrocarbon burns completely, it releases carbon dioxide and water, while liberating the solar energy used to form it. Burning or oxidizing literally reverses the energy process begun by the sun. The amount of energy released, as calories of heat, is directly related to the amount of oxygen used for the process. That is the reason scientists can measure the amount of oxygen you consume and know rather accurately how many calories your body is releasing. This relationship is based on the most fundamental laws of energy.

Such information has even been of value in planning manned space

---

*Strictly speaking a hydrocarbon contains only carbon and hydrogen. Carbohydrates also contain oxygen, fat contains very little oxygen and proteins contain very little oxygen and some nitrogen in addition to carbon and hydrogen.

flights. The amount of oxygen that astronauts will require for a given number of hours or days in space depends on how much energy they must use. That tells the space scientists how much oxygen must be transported with the space vehicle.

Discovering Oxygen

One of the first demonstrations that fire and metabolism were similar was done as early at 1669 by John Mayow, British physiologist. Oxygen hadn't even been discovered yet. His ingenious experiment had three parts. First, he put a mouse on a platform in water. Then he placed a glass chamber over the mouse and the water. The mouse was literally trapped on the platform in an air bubble. He noted that as the mouse lived, the water rose in the glass chamber. That was because the mouse was using oxygen to process food. The second part of the experiment was to put a lighted candle on the platform instead of the mouse. As the candle burned, the water rose in the glass chamber. Again, it was for the same reason. The flame of the candle used the oxygen in the air for combustion. Finally, he placed both the mouse and a candle under a glass chamber. The mouse only lived about half as long. Why? Because the candle used part of the available oxygen.

It remained for Joseph Priestley, a British scientist, to make pure oxygen by heating potassium nitrate (niter or salt peter, the substance falsely claimed to decrease the sex drive in males), which released oxygen. He observed that a mouse lived much longer using the same volume of this new gas than when breathing ordinary air.

A noted French scientist, Antione Laurent Lavoisier, who lived in the 18th century, was the father of modern chemistry. He was the first to observe the relationship between oxygen and heat energy. He recognized that foods were like fuels and were composed of hydrogen, carbon and oxygen. He established that oxidation of foods and fuels to carbon dioxide and water produced a predictable amount of heat. By demonstrating this, he provided the first basis for the relationship of oxygen to calories of heat energy produced.

The Law of Conservation of Energy

In those early days of chemistry and physics, the great brains of the time were still unlocking the basic secrets of energy. As recently as

1842, an English physicist, James Prestcott Joule, established that mechanical energy was equivalent to heat energy. An example of mechanical energy is the amount of energy required to move your car one block. In physics, this is all related to units of work. To keep it simple, remember that one unit used to measure work is the joule, so named after the English physicist. From Joule's work came a fundamental relationship that one calorie of heat was equal to 4.18 joules. You don't need to remember that, but you do need to know that there is a direct relationship between mechanical energy and heat energy or calories.

Also in 1842, a German physician, Julius Robert von Mayer, published a revolutionary theory that was to become the basis for understanding energy on our planet, and indeed, in the universe. Basically, he stated that the total amount of energy in the universe remained constant, but any one form of energy, such as calories of heat, could be converted to another form of energy, such as joules of mechanical energy.

You probably don't think about this when you flip on the light switch and, behold, electrical energy is converted to light energy. If you touch the light bulb, you will find it is also producing heat energy. Your electric oven is a good example of converting electrical energy to heat energy. When you run the vacuum cleaner, you are converting electrical energy to mechanical energy. The von Mayer theory encompassed the idea that electrical energy could be converted to heat energy or mechanical energy. Electrical energy, thermal energy, mechanical energy, chemical energy—all were just expressions of the total energy in the universe, and any one form of energy could be converted to the other.

It remained for another famous German scientist, Hermann von Helmholtz, to use this theory to formulate one of the basic laws of nature, called the Law of Conservation of Energy. I can't overemphasize the importance of this simple law to help you understand what your body does with food energy. The law states simply, *Energy can neither be created nor destroyed.*

Think about that a minute. It means there is no magical way you can eliminate calories. Every speck of energy must be accounted for. Remember, I said that your body did not use calories, but was an energy converter. It converts the calories of energy in your food to heat, to mechanical energy, to chemical energy, or it stores energy as body fat. Body fat is stored hydrocarbon. It is your energy bank. But your body does not destroy or use up calories. You can account for what happens to every single calorie of energy that enters your body. Calories do count. The basis for that fundamental truth rests on the basic laws of nature established by these early giants of the middle 19th century. That does not mean you cannot influence how your body converts calories. Of course you can, but your body will only do this in accordance with fundamental laws that no one can change. Many false claims about fad diets ignore this fundamental law of nature. Since many people do not understand this fundamental truth, they become victims of such false claims.

Measuring Food Calories

The number of calories of energy that are in your food can be measured directly. That is done by using an ingenious device called the bomb calorimeter. Have you ever wondered how it was determined how many calories were in a gram of carbohydrate, a gram of protein or a gram of fat? Max Rubner, and others who followed him, used the bomb calorimeter to do this. He measured the number of calories of heat produced by burning various foods inside a metal chamber, called a bomb. The item to be measured is completely burned inside the bomb. A specific measure of the food is placed inside the bomb, which is then loaded with pure oxygen. The food is then ignited with an electric spark. The heat produced by the complete combustion of the food in the metal chamber is transferred to a measured amount of water surrounding it. From the change in termperature of the water, the calories of heat produced by burning the food can be measured. In this way, early studies provided the measures in common use today, that one gram of carbohydrate contains 4 calories, one gram of protein 4 calories and one gram of fat 9 calories. This is a slight generalization, but it is sufficiently accurate for practical use. These early studies also established how much oxygen was used to release the calories in carbohydrates, proteins and fat.

You might ask if the calories in your food will react the same way in your body. They do. Rubner used another chamber to measure the heat given off by the body. He fed some of the same foods that were burned in the bomb calorimeter to a dog. Then he measured the amount of heat that was liberated from the dog's body. He found that the amount of heat energy released from the dog's body was equal to the amount

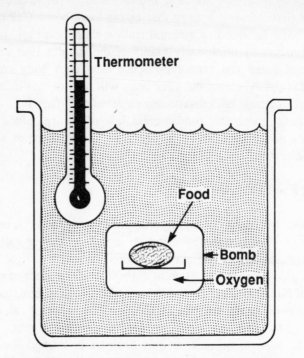

Oxygen used to burn food releases calories that heat the water. The heat is measured by a thermometer. This is how calories in carbohydrates, proteins, fat and various foods have been measured.

of heat liberated from the same food placed in the bomb calorimeter.

Those were important early studies. Note that the first real studies of the energy in foods were related to measuring the heat produced by the food and by the body. These early studies also established another point that is very important to you—the energy you consume is normally released from your body as heat. Almost all the energy that leaves your body at rest is as heat, and that means most of it must be liberated through your skin. A small amount is lost as heat through your lungs. Also, a small amount of energy is lost in the urea and eliminated in the urine. The urea is formed to eliminate excess nitrogen from the breakdown of protein, but this is of little importance in eliminating calories.

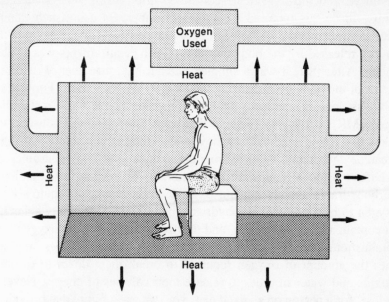

The calories of heat produced by a person depends on the amount of oxygen used. At rest, the calories of heat produced equals the calories a person uses. You can measure the oxygen used and calculate the calories used.

Your skin is the most important portal of exit for calories leaving your body. You probably never thought about your skin being important in the weighting game, but it is one of the most significant factors in controlling your calorie balance. The fundamental fact that energy leaves the body as heat is why the calorie was used as a convenient measure for energy exchange by the body. When you think of calories, think of heat, heat in your hydrocarbon foods and heat liberated from your body.

These early experiments firmly established that the combustion of food released a specific amount of heat. They also demonstrated that this required a specific amount of oxygen for the amount of heat released. Once the relationship between calories of heat produced and oxygen was established, the next step was to study the relationship between calories in food, calories of heat produced and oxygen used in man. This was done in a device that both measured the heat a man produced and the oxygen he consumed after eating measured food items. To do this required a complex chamber. By using such chambers, a fundamental relationship between energy in food, calories of energy released by the body and the oxygen requirements was established. After that, it was a simple matter to measure energy requirements of the body by measuring the oxygen the body used. For years, this was done in medical practice by measuring the basal metabolic rate (BMR). I'll say more about that later, but for now it is useful to know that if you need to know how many calories your body is using, it can be determined by measuring the oxygen your body consumes.

Different foods require different amounts of oxygen for oxidation. Carbohydrates already contain oxygen. As a result, it requires less oxygen to break down carbohydrates than other foods. Fatty acids in fat contain almost no oxygen, and they require much more oxygen for combustion. The oxygen in amino acids from protein varies, and so does the amount of oxygen required to break them down to carbon dioxide and water in order to release their calories of energy. Nevertheless, for a person on a mixed diet, you can use a figure that provides a useful measure of the energy being exchanged. That figure is 4.825. For every liter of oxygen your body is using, it is using 4.825 calories. If you are resting, and your body uses only 15 liters of oxygen an hour, that would mean your body is using 1,737 calories a day just for resting requirements (15 liters x 24 hours = 360 liters; 360 x 4.825 calories = 1,737 calories). Incidentally, that figure is well within the range seen in an average-sized male. The practical point is that if you can get your oxygen consumption at rest measured, it can be used to calculate about how many calories a day your body would use at rest. That figure can be important in knowing how many calories should be in your daily diet.

Would you like to know how much energy a physically fit astronaut can use during maximum exertion? When my colleagues and I examined the Gemini and Apollo astronauts we measured their total oxygen consumption when they had reached their maximum physical effort. As an example, Astronaut Ed White, the first astronaut to walk in space, used 4,737 ml of oxygen a minute at maximum exertion. His heart rate was 200 beats a minute. That means he used 22.856 calories a minute or equivalent to 1,371 calories an hour (4.737 liters x 4.825 calories = 22.856 calories; 22.856 calories per minute x 60 minutes

= 1,371 calories). Of course people can only sustain these high levels of energy output for a short period of time.

Basal Metabolic Rate (BMR)

Shortly after investigators began measuring the amount of oxygen a person used to calculate the calories a person needed, it became apparent that the measurements didn't correlate well with the subject's weight. Oxygen use did correlate much better with the body surface area. A heavy, round object has less surface area than a flat object of the same weight and same material. Expressing the results in terms of body surface area refined the measurements somewhat. The body surface area was calculated from a subject's height and weight and expressed in square meters. Studies showed that normal men between the ages of 25 and 50 used from 37 to 40 calories per square meter of body surface area per hour, under basal conditions. A man of average height and weight will have a body surface area of about 1.95 square meters. Using 38 calories per square meter of body surface area per hour, that means he would use 74.1 calories an hour or 1,778 calories under basal conditions over a 24-hour period. Deviations from the normal value were expressed in terms of percentage. That is how the BMR came to be expressed as plus or minus a percentage, such as plus 10 percent, plus 20 percent, or minus 15 percent of the expected value.

The requirement to do the test under basal conditions made this quite a ritual. The subject to be tested was to be as quiet as possible without being asleep during the test. He was asked to eat only a very light evening meal no later than 7:00 P.M. the evening before testing. He was to get a good night's sleep and report to the facility. I recall in my early days in medicine that in the early morning hours—before the other patients arrived—the clinic rooms were filled with sleepy patients having their BMR tested. The tests were to be done 12 to 14 hours after the evening meal, or around 9:00 A.M. The testing was done in a quiet, dimly lighted room after the subject had rested quietly in the room for at least 30 minutes. The results of the test were based on how much oxygen the subject used while in this basal state. As you have seen from the earlier studies, the oxygen consumed could be used to calculate the calories of energy the subject was using in that basal state.

These tests were very popular because at that time they were the only way to really assess thyroid function. They were really used as a thyroid test. Their great value in assessing how many calories the body needed, and using that figure as a basis of evaluating a subject's nutritional requirements, was largely ignored. That is unfortunate because noting the oxygen consumption from that same procedure would be invaluable in determining a patient's actual calorie use and calorie needs. For every liter of oxygen the subject uses, he is using about 4.825 calories at rest. Even worse, because the oxygen consumption measured metabolism, regardless of what affected the metabolism, the BMR was not a very reliable measure of thyroid function. It was an excellent test used for the wrong reason.

Eventually, much more accurate and direct tests of thyroid function were developed. When this occurred, it became apparent how inaccurate the BMR often was as a measure of thyroid function. However, measuring thyroid functions with these new tests does not measure a person's metabolism, only thyroid function. Energy requirements depend on much more than just thyroid function. The end result was that the BMR test nearly passed out of existence. Today, oxygen consumption measurements are more commonly used as part of measuring how much blood the heart pumps or in evaluating lung function.

Even light muscular activity will increase the metabolism. Just the effort involved in getting dressed may raise the metabolism 25 to 60 percent above basal levels. But those who get tired from mental work will be surprised to learn that one hour of intense mental work will increase the metabolism so little that the requirements can be met with one-half of a salted peanut.

Calories for Fat-Free Body

One of the problems with the BMR is that it was expressed in terms of a square meter of body surface area. The tables used for this are not that accurate. When two people of nearly the same height are tested, and one is fat but the other is not, the value is apt to be distorted because of the increased amount of body fat. Since many people gain body fat as they get older, this led to the belief that as you got older, "the metabolic fires burned ever slower."

In fact, the metabolism does not slow down as you get older. Dr. Ancel Keys' group at the University of Minnesota measured the oxygen consumption in people of different ages and with different amounts of body fat. They used the weight of the body minus the body fat, which they called the fat-free body weight. They found that the energy requirements in relationship to fat-free body weight were rather constant, despite wide variations in the BMR. If you don't try to manipulate the calories used in relation to body surface area, the oxygen consumption is a very good measure of the energy used by the fat-free body weight. They even found it was fairly constant for both men and women between the ages of 20 and 60.

These normal people used about 4.4 ml of oxygen per minute per kilogram of fat-free body weight, under basal conditions. That may be expressed as 1.28 calories per hour per kilogram (2.2 pounds) of body weight. Your metabolically active tissues, such as muscles, do not use less energy as you get older. But people do tend to get fatter and have less muscle weight. That is why the amount of oxygen they need decreases, not because the metabolism of the active tissues is slowed.

Summary 2

1. A food calorie is the amount of heat energy required to increase the temperature of 1,000 ml (1 liter) of water 1 degree Centigrade.
2. Oxygen is required to "metabolize" or burn food to release calories of heat energy.
3. The amount of oxygen you use exactly measures the amount of energy your body uses.
4. Any form of energy can be converted to another form of energy— for example, electrical energy may be converted to mechanical energy or heat energy.
5. Nature's law of conservation of energy states, "Energy can neither be created nor destroyed." Food energy, and what your body does with it, must conform to this fundamental law of nature.
6. The amount of oxygen required to metabolize your food is a direct measure of the amount of energy in calories of heat in your food. The measurement of heat produced and oxygen used is how the number of calories in carbohydrates, fats, proteins and alcohol has been determined.

Chapter 3

Controlling Your Metabolic Furnace

You may think that you control your appetite, but that is not entirely so. Some people really do have an overwhelming urge to eat. Others have a rather small appetite. Many factors will determine just how strong that urge to eat really is. Your brain evidently encourages your body to eat enough to maintain a proper calorie balance, unless you are ill, then the brain may respond to signals that suggest you shouldn't eat, or, as we say, you lose your appetite.

The Brain Controls

One of the most striking indications of the influence of the brain over appetite is how it causes hypothalamic obesity. The hypothalamus is literally the floor of the mid-brain region. It is just above the roof of your mouth. I like to think of this area as the switchboard for the signals entering the brain. Your thermostat is located here. It senses your body temperature, and it is directly related to your emotions. It is connected to your sympathetic nervous system (part of your involuntary nervous system) that governs much of the automatic activity in your body. The cells that control your appetite are located here, also. For years it has been known that if you damage a specific area within the hypothalamus, you can cause an animal to get fat. The same thing happens to a human if that area of the brain is injured. This doesn't cause a person to get fat as if by magic. Rather, the person starts eating more than usual, and that excess calorie intake results in hypothalamic obesity.

25

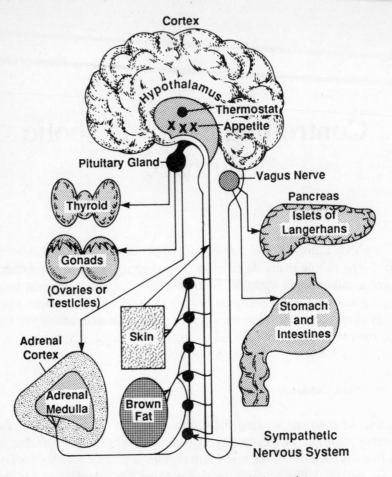

The brain controls calorie balance through:
1) Its control of the major endocrine glands
2) The sympathetic nervous system and hypothalamus
3) The vagus nerve from the brain stem

Specific cells in your brain control the function of various parts of your body. You have cells that stimulate the movement of your arm. If these cells are damaged by a stroke, your arm will be paralyzed. A similar system exists for many other functions of the body, including functions that affect your appetite. When insulin is released from your pancreas, that causes your blood glucose to fall, and stimulates the appetite center in your brain. The vagus nerve from your brain, which goes to most of the organs and structures in your abdomen and chest, can stimulate the pancreas to release insulin. You can prevent hypothalamic obesity by simply cutting the vagus nerve fibers to the pancreas. Or you can destroy the islets of Langerhans in the pancreas that form insulin so this won't happen. It appears that hypothalamic obesity is related to an increased production of insulin.

The appetite center may not be a center after all. At one time, scientists thought there was one appetite center that stimulated eating, and another than inhibited the appetite center. New concepts of brain chemistry suggest that, rather than localized centers, there may be specialized nerve cells that have this function. These calls are sensitive to certain chemicals. The details of the nerve fibers and receptors remain to be established, but we do know that the brain, "your little black box," does stimulate you to eat, and even affects how much you eat of what. Your brain literally determines how much energy you will consume. You can think of it as how much metabolic fuel is being loaded into your metabolic chamber to be fired with oxygen and release calories of heat as energy. In a sense, you are a biological bomb calorimeter.

How can you influence your brain's appetite controls? One of the important factors is the amount of glucose (sugar) in your blood. Your brain seems to be sensitive to the difference in the amount of glucose in your arterial blood as compared to your venous blood. It is interesting to note that your brain normally uses glucose exclusively as its source of energy, so it is especially sensitive to your blood glucose level. As your blood glucose level falls, or the difference between the amount of glucose in your arteries and your veins changes, the appetite function is stimulated. Your brain cortex, the conscious part of your brain, starts getting signals that you need to eat, and soon you have an overwhelming desire to eat. When you do, and the blood glucose rises, the sensation of hunger disappears. Mothers have long used this fact by asking their children not to eat candy or other sweets before a meal, because, "it will spoil your appetite."

Your Stretch Receptors

Nerve receptors in your digestive system also send signals to your appetite control cells. Your stomach and intestines may be empty and start rhythmic contractions, or hunger pains. When your stomach is full, the stimulus to eat is turned off. Many diets depend on this aspect of appetite control to help people limit their calorie intake. Foods that provide lots of bulk, but contain few usable calories, fill the stomach and turn off the appetite. There are also receptors that detect the acidity in the stomach and detect what is happening in your intestines. All of this is relayed to your appetite controls in your brain.

The stretch receptors in the stomach provide the basis for some new approaches to controlling calorie intake. One of these is stapling the stomach.. By limiting the size of the stomach pouch to store food, the stretch fibers are stimulated earlier. This means the individual feels full after eating less. A similar effect is produced by putting an inflated balloon in the stomach. That inflated balloon means it takes less food to stimulate the stretch receptors. Again, the appetite control system gets the signal that the stomach is full, and you can stop eating.

The appetite system is not totally dependent upon signals from the digestive system. This has been demonstrated by experiments on animals that involved cutting the nerve fibers to the entire digestive system. Despite this, the animals continued to eat normally without either gaining or losing weight.

Your Conditioned Responses

Conditioned responses are among the most important factors to stimulate your appetite control system. Since we have a habit of regulating our lives, and eating at specific times, we get hungry at that time whether we need calories or not. Such a conditioned response was demonstrated by the famous Russian physiologist, Ivan Pavlov. He constructed a pouch to a dog's stomach so he could measure the onset and amount of digestive juices secreted by the stomach. Then he observed that the onset of feeding caused an outpouring of digestive juices. The next step was to ring a bell every time the dog was given food. Soon, he was able to ring the bell and the digestive juices would start flowing. Any of the things that we have learned through time to associate with eating cause us to have conditioned responses. If you eat at noon, as the noon hour approaches you will begin to feel hungry.

Your appetite control system does respond to many different cues. Just seeing your favorite food may make you hungry. An attractive dining room, a roaring fire and a well-set table laden with your favorite foods are sure to stimulate your appetite. The smell of coffee brewing in the morning may be the cue that starts your digestive juices flowing. Drinking a cup of coffee with a friend, or in a social setting, may become almost a conditioned response.

It is sometimes hard to separate psychological from social factors that stimulate your appetite. It is clear that psychological factors are an important part of stimulating some people to eat. A person may literally have had behavioral training to eat under certain circumstances. A good example is providing food as a reward. When a child is rewarded with his favorite food or candy for certain achievements or behavior, he tends to associate those foods with rewards. Later, when he is able to do so, he may reward himself with those foods. The reward concept extends further, to celebrating with a good meal because you deserved it. How many times have you celebrated some event in your life by splurging on food?

A Matter of Chemistry

Rewards are not the only psychological aspect of eating. Some people eat because of boredom. Others eat because they are depressed. Oddly, other people stop eating because they are depressed. Since depression is closely related to brain chemistry, and brain chemistry affects appetite, it is not surprising to see a correlation between depression and eating.

Depression may occur because of a depletion of norepinephrine in the brain. Norepinephrine, also called noradrenaline, is normally produced at the many points where one sympathetic nerve fiber meets another. It enables the transmission of impulses from the end of one nerve fiber to another. A very closely related chemical, adrenaline, is formed mostly by the center of the adrenal gland, and is released into your bloodstream when you are under stress.

Adrenaline (epinephrine) is transmitted mainly by your circulation while noradrenaline is mostly involved with your sympathetic nervous system. However, some adrenaline is present in your nerve fiber action, and the center of your adrenal gland does release some noradrenaline. When norephinephrine is delivered to specific cells in your hypothalamus, it stimulates you to eat. Thus, replacing the norepinephrine in the brain may lift your depression and stimulate your appetite so that you gain weight. This is also a good example to point out what can happen in your body. Two things can and do happen without one of them causing the other one. The norepinephrine does not just lift your depression, and then because you are no longer depressed you start eating. The norepinephrine can do both, lift your depression and simultaneously increase your appetite by stimulating your appetite control system.

Norepinephrine is called a monamine. Another important monamine in depression is serotonin. When your brain is depleted of serotonin, you will become depressed. One class of medicines used to treat depressions have their effect by helping restore the monamines in the brain. Serotonin also helps to transmit impulses between nerve fibers in your brain. These mechanisms gave rise to a recent theory about why people have a strong urge to eat sweets.

The theory, popularized by Judith Wurtman, Ph.D. at Massachusetts Institute of Technology, is based on the movement of amino acids. Remember that the protein in your food is made up of amino acids. There is a pool of these in your blood and body fluids, called the amino acid pool. But these cannot get into your brain very easily. We have a blood-brain barrier which keeps many of them from passing from your circulation into your brain cells. Only a few of the large number of amino acids can get through at a time. It is much like a busy 12-lane freeway, loaded with cars, ending in one narrow traffic lane. The various amino acids compete with each other to get through that barrier. One of these amino acids, tryptophan, is converted by your brain into serotonin. If it can get into the brain, it can raise your brain serotonin level.

What do sweets have to do with getting tryptophan into your brain? Sweets cause your pancreas to release insulin. The insulin enhances the movement of certain amino acids into your muscles. It is like opening up a detour off the 12-lane freeway that siphons off most of the automobiles, except the tryptophan sports cars. Since there is less competition, the tryptophan moves easily through the limited access and enters the brain cells. In this way, sweets enhance the tryptophan content of the brain, which in turn raises the serotonin level in the brain. As the serotonin level rises, the appetite urge for sweets subsides, and a person's mood lifts. It is a neat theory, and may explain part of the picture, but don't forget that a rise in blood glucose alone may help to turn off your appetite.

Some doctors have used an appetite suppressant, Pondimin

(fenfluramine), to help people lose weight. This medicine may help to build up the serotonin level in the brain. It is not a brain stimulant, as many appetite suppressants are. It may actually make you sleepy. Unfortunately, you can develop a physical dependence on this medication.

Changing your body chemistry in various ways can suppress your appetite. This happens with many illnesses. A person with significant changes in liver function may lose his appetite. Many toxins that are released during infectious illnesses may have this effect. The effects of chemical imbalance is the basis for the low-carbohydrate diets decreasing a person's appetite. They cause an overproduction of ketones, the same chemicals produced when a diabetic is out of control and going into diabetic acidosis and coma. Starvation results in the same chemical changes. After an initial period of one to three days, the starving person may no longer have the urge to eat.

Your Thyroid Stimulates Burning

Once food fuel is delivered to your digestive system, it must then be digested and absorbed into your circulation before it can be combusted to release energy. It is the same as the requirement to have fuel in the furnace before it can be burned to release heat. Food combustion actually takes place within your cells. That includes your liver, brain, kidneys, heart, all other organs, and, of course, your muscles. Cells do not survive without a source of energy, and that energy must come from food, or from fat and glycogen stores that were previously formed from food energy. As the combustion takes place, calories of heat are released. Some of these are used to maintain your body temperature. If that goal is met, then the rest must be eliminated or your body temperature will rise progressively, and you will have a heat stroke. The process of burning your absorbed foods to release energy is part of your metabolism.

Your thyroid gland, which is ultimately controlled by your brain, releases thyroid hormone (thyroxine) which stimulates cellular metabolism. If you do not produce enough thyroxine, you are said to have a low metabolism. When you produce an excess of thyroxine, you have an increased metabolism. The thyroid gland plays an important role in burning your food to provide your energy. When you are not getting enough to eat, your thyroid function is literally decreased, lowering your metabolism. This is nature's way of protecting you from starvation. If your metabolism is lower, you don't need so much energy, and you can survive longer. Your stores of body fat, which is stored energy, last longer. That is great if you are in a survival situation, but frustrating if you want to lose some extra pounds of body fat. Actually, a major mechanism to lower metabolism is to change thyroid hormone into a form that will not stimulate metabolism. This occurs outside the thyroid gland in the body tissues. The inactive thyroid hormone is called reverse thyroxin (rT3). Since this change in the hormone is accomplished after the thyroid hormone has been released from the thyroid gland, the gland's function may be normal when tested. But, the active form of thyroid hormone that stimulates metabolism is diminished, lowering metabolism. That is a good example why measuring oxygen consumption is not always a good measure of the thyroid gland's function.

The changes in function of the thyroid gland in response to diet again demonstrate that your body has many mechanisms to try to keep you at a steady weight. It helps to explain why some people can eat and not gain weight, while others decrease their calories and do not lose weight. If a normal person overeats for three to four weeks, the thyroid gland produces more hormone, and the person's metabolism is raised. The increased metabolism prevent him from gaining body fat. The increase in metabolism associated with overfeeding is comparable to the decrease in metabolism observed when a person is underfed. There is a lesson in this for you about your energy level, too. If you are eating properly, and not suffering from undernutrition, your metabolism will be regulated at the proper level. An increased calorie intake actually will increase your metabolism and your level of energy.

Those carbohydrate-free diets that have been so popular affect the thyroid gland. The amount of usable thyroid hormone decreases, just as it does in starvation, causing the metabolism to decrease. So does a person's energy. But carbohydrates can increase the metabolism in humans. If you replace, calorie for calorie, a major portion of the diet with carbohydrates, you can increase the production of thyroid hormone to mimic that produced by overfeeding. That is a sound basis for using a high-carbohydrate diet rather than a low-carbohydrate diet, if you are on a diet to eliminate body fat and don't want to be fatigued.

Exposure to cold increases your metabolism. When you are exposed to cold, the stress stimulates the release of adrenaline. The adrenaline increases metabolism and generates heat. That is an emergency measure. In rat experiments, it has been shown that exposure to cold for three weeks caused the metabolism to rise as much as 16 percent. There is also an increase in the size of the thyroid gland. This effect, too, is mediated through the brain. The thyroid gland is regulated by the pituitary gland, located under your brain. If the stem-like connection between the pituitary gland and the hypothalamus under the brain is cut, the increase in metabolism from cold exposure does not occur. Even the action of adrenaline to increase metabolism requires thyroid hormone. If the thyroid gland is removed, the increased heat production normally induced by adrenaline does not occur.

Brown Fat in the Fire

Thyroid hormone stimulates your body cells to increase their metabolic action, and this releases heat. There is a second way the body can increase the release of calories, and it is from fat cells, a process that can help you stay lean. Yes, that is right, fat cells that may help you stay lean instead of getting fat. This seeming paradox is based on the observation that there are two types of fat cells. The type you have heard about most of the time is white or yellow fat. That makes up the majority of fat under your skin and around your organs. It is the type of fat that many people would like to eliminate, if they could.

There is another type of cells that contain "brown fat." They are very unusual fat cells as they contain the machinery to burn fat rapidly to release calories. Brown fat cells are well supplied with sympathetic nerve fibers. The nerve fibers release norepinephrine, which stimulates the process. White fat cells don't have the same type of nerve supply and are actually storage depots for fat, until such time as it is mobilized and taken elsewhere to be burned to provide energy.

In animals, brown fat is an important mechanism in keeping the animal warm. It is abundant in animals that must survive in cold climates. It is scattered throughout the body, particularly in the chest, around the heart and in the thorax, under the scapula (shoulder blade) in the axilla (arm pit areas) and scattered throughout the abdomen. When the animal is stressed by cold, the sympathetic nerve fibers release noradrenaline and stimulate the brown fat cells to start burning fat, which releases calories of heat. Epinephrine and insulin, arriving at the cells by the circulation, also stimulate the brown fat cells.

There are two different factors that stimulate the brown fat cells. One is cold. The other is consuming food, particularly if the animal is being overfed. Brown fat, then, helps to stabilize the animal's temperature and also helps to stabilize his weight. If he eats too much, the brown fat simply releases a lot more calories of heat, which are then eliminated from the body. This helps to explain why many animals under free-living conditions, with adequate food, tend to maintain the same weight, despite significant changes in their pattern of food intake.

Do you have brown fat? Probably. For some time, there was considerable doubt that humans had any significant amounts of brown fat. Indeed, brown fat is less abundant in all mammals than in other animals. It has now been demonstrated that brown fat is abundant in newborn infants, and although it is hard to identify, its characteristics have been noted at all ages. Tests measuring the temperatures of different surface areas of the skin have identified hot spots that seem to be related to underlying brown fat. Also, it has been demonstrated that exposure of both adults and infants to cold will stimulate the sympathetic nerves and speeds up metabolism. This suggests the existence of brown fat.

The amount of brown fat in humans has been estimated by injecting norepinephrine and measuring the change in metabolism. Metabolism increases from 30 to 60 percent. That increase is a measure of what you can expect from brown fat cells in terms of converting fat to calories of heat. That is a lot less than the 300 percent increase in metabolism noted in many animals when injected with norepinephrine. Nevertheless, it is effective.

How cold does it have to be to cause brown fat to start releasing calories of heat? Exposure to 22 degrees C (72 degrees F) stimulates the sympathetic nerve response and will significantly speed up metabolism at rest.

The response of brown fat cells to eating is a lot more difficult to assess. We do know that sympathetic nerve activity decreases when you fast and increases when you eat. These changes are associated with an increase in metabolism after eating. Just overeating for one day will increase metabolism for as long as 12 hours after the last meal. If you feel hot after eating a big meal, your increased metabolism is the reason.

What is the relationship between your thyroid gland and brown fat?

It appears that thyroid hormone is necessary to enable brown fat cells to burn fat, although it doesn't participate in the brown fat's action. Actually, they complement each other. If your cells are stimulated by thyroid hormone, and produce lots of heat in the process, then brown fat activity slows or ceases to exist. Anything you do that increases the body's temperature seems to stop the action of brown fat. It is likely that a person who starves, but manages to stay warm, will not have much brown fat action. On the contrary, the person who is exposed to cold, and eats a lot, will have active, well-developed brown fat that serves to keep his body temperature up and his body fat stores down. A good example of this is the observation that brown fat develops around the neck of outdoor workers in Finland.

It is possible that emotional stress may stimulate brown fat action. Many people sweat when they are under emotional stress. Part of that may be from an increased action of brown fat cells, caused by the sympathetic nerve fibers releasing norepinephrine, and the actions of epinephrine. Emotional stress causes a release of these hormones. This offers a plausible explanation of how people under emotional stress lose weight, even though they are eating normally. Their bodies are geared to increasing the release of calories of heat.

There have been some interesting observations about inherited defects in brown fat cell function in rats and mice that may have a bearing on obesity in some humans. At the very least, it documents one of the ways obesity can be inherited. One strain of laboratory mice that are obese while on a regular cafeteria diet have no ability to withstand cold. They will die if they are exposed to temperatures of 4 degrees C for even a few hours. They are unable to turn on brown fat cells to release calories of heat. They are fat and cold because of an inherited defect in their brown fat cells. It is quite possible that some people who are overweight, and also feel cold, have a defect in their brown fat cell mechanism that is comparable to that in these mice.

Zucker rats are a fat strain of rats. They get fat on the same diets that normal lean control rats eat. They can withstand cold because their brown fat cells generate the needed heat to respond to cold stress, but they do not respond to the stimulus of eating by releasing calories of heat. The Zucker rats inherit a defect in their thermal response to eating. They may have a counterpart in people who inherit a similar defect and do not increase their heat production when they eat. The end result is obesity.

The type of food a person eats may affect one's metabolism. Normally, there is an increase in metabolism after eating. But, just as Zucker rats are different from other rats, the same seems to be true for some overweight people compared to lean people. A study recently reported showed that lean individuals and fat individuals had a similar increase in metabolism after being given glucose or protein, but there was no increase in metabolism in fat subjects after ingesting fat (*American Journal of Clinical Nutrition*, August 1985). Since a gram of fat contains 9 calories, it follows that the failure to show an increase in metabolism after ingesting fat can only mean that these calories were retained by the body. At this time, there is no explanation for this difference between lean and fat individuals, but it is worth thinking about if you are overweight and want to eliminate body fat. It suggests that you should avoid fat in your diet.

Summary 3

Factors That Affect Appetite
1. Certain brain injuries or defects may stimulate an increase in appetite.
2. As the blood glucose level falls, the appetite is stimulated. When it rises, the appetite is diminished.
3. Stretch receptors in the stomach and the rest of the digestive system affect appetite. When the stomach is full these reflexes inhibit the appetite. When the digestive system is empty, that stimulates the appetite.
4. Conditioned responses and various cues may stimulate appetite. One of the best examples is feeling hungry, "because it is time to eat." Visual cues, smells or thoughts may stimulate the appetite.
5. Psychological factors stimulate the appetite. This includes the habit of receiving food rewards for various reasons. Boredom may result in eating.
6. Depression is associated with chemical changes in the brain — the neurotransmitters — that can either stimulate the appetite or decrease the appetite.
7. Brain chemicals affect your appetite. These include norepinephrine (noradrenaline) and low serotonin levels. These are called neurotransmitters because they are essential to the function of nerve impulses in the brain.

8. Toxins from various illnesses may decrease a person's appetite.
9. Eliminating carbohydrates or starvation results in forming ketones which decreases the appetite.

Factors That Affect Release of Calories of Heat
1. When the thyroid gland produces an excess of thyroid hormone (thyroxine), it stimulates cell metabolism and increases the release of calories of heat.
2. When the thyroid gland fails to produce enough hormone, cell metabolism decreases and the calories of heat produced decreases.
3. When you don't consume enough calories, thyroid hormone is inactivated, decreasing metabolism and decreasing the release of calories of heat. Your energy system is slowed down.
4. Eating more carbohydrates in place of fat stimulates thyroid action.
5. Adrenaline stimulates cell metabolism. It is released when you are exposed to cold to stimulate the cells to release more calories of heat. Thyroid hormone is essential for this response to cold to occur.
6. There is a special form of fat, called brown fat, that burns fat to produce heat.
7. Brown fat activity to release calories of heat is stimulated by both cold exposure and by eating an excessive amount of calories. Brown fat is one of the mechanisms that helps to stabilize weight despite variations in calorie intake.
8. Emotional stress, through the release of noradrenaline, stimulates brown fat and may be one mechanism of weight loss from stress.
9. Inherited defects in certain animals prevent normal brown fat action to release calories and may be one cause of obesity.

Chapter 4

Eliminating Calories of Heat

The weighting game has usually focused on the number of calories people consume and the energy involved in physical activity. It is very surprising that scant attention has been paid to how the body eliminates calories. Since body fat is stored calories, it is fairly obvious that the amount of fat stored is related to both the number of calories consumed and the number of calories eliminated. The whole basis of the calorie balance and body fat equation is simply stated as:

Calories consumed − Calories used = Calories stored as body fat.

An important half of this fundamental equation, how the body loses calories, has been largely ignored. You might say that is why people exercise and count the calories needed for exercise, but that is just a small part of the calories that your body eliminates. The problem is far more complicated than running a mile, or a weekly session at your aerobics class. You are eliminating calories every second, whether you are sitting, sleeping, watching TV or running around the block. Almost all of your calories are eliminated from your body as heat, and nearly all of those calories of heat are eliminated through your skin. Remember the analogy I gave you at the beginning—your body is like a large room, with a furnace at one end and an air conditioner at the other end. Your skin is your air conditioner. It cools your body. That means it eliminates calories. Whenever your metabolic fires are turned up, your skin has to eliminate more calories to prevent your body temperature from climbing. And when you are exposed to cold, and lose calories through your skin, your metabolic furnace must be turned up to keep your body temperature from falling. The heat-loss mechanism through your skin is important to your weight balance, and it is controlled by your brain.

Your skin has four main ways of eliminating calories; by radiation, conduction, convection and evaporation. Heat literally radiates from your body surface. Whenever you stand near something that has a lower temperature than you do, heat leaves your body and is absorbed by that object. If you were standing next to something that is warmer than your body, you would tend to absorb radiant heat. When you warm yourself at an open fire, you absorb radiant heat. About half of the calories eliminated by your body each day are as radiant heat. Clothing will trap this radiant heat and diminish the heat loss. At the same time, clothing will protect you from radiant heat from the sun, and prevent your body from trapping the sun's radiant heat. You feel cooler standing in the shade than in the sun because you are partially protected from the sun's radiation.

If you are tall and thin, that may help you avoid gaining pounds of fat. A tall, thin person has a larger amount of body surface area than another person who is of the same weight but shorter and heavier. Because the tall, thin person constantly loses more calories by radiation, he can consume more calories than his short, stocky counterpart without getting fat. It is a vicious cycle. If you are short and stocky, you are likely to get heavier, but if you are tall and thin, you are likely to stay that way.

Almost all of the skin's surface loses calories through radiation. The exceptions are the areas where opposing surfaces of the skin prevent exposure, such as under the arms. But nature has compensated for this by increasing the number of sweat glands in those locations. There is a reason why people are more likely to sweat under the arms.

There is also a reason why a person tends to curl up when he is cold. That curled position decreases the amount of skin surface that is exposed, and he feels warmer. It is probably true that if people went naked, they would have less of a problem with being overweight (for many reasons), but that is not a viable option in our society.

Conduction of heat means the transfer of calories from one object to another through direct contact. One of the best examples is to get into a pool of cold water. Heat immediately flows from the skin surface to the cold water. Water is a fairly good conductor so you can lose a lot of heat that way. Conversely, if you are in a hot tub of water with a temperature greater than your skin, calories will be conducted to the skin's surface. Air is a poor conductor so at room temperature you normally lose only 2 or 3 percent of calories through conduction. Various substances have different capacities to conduct heat. A poor conductor such as air actually is an insulator. In fact the way much of the insulation in houses work is by trapping pockets of air. Clothing is a poor conductor and insulates the body. Fat, under the skin, will not prevent the skin from working as your air conditioner, but it will act as insulation to prevent direct transfer of heat from the body organs and muscles to the skin and out the body.

Your body eliminates another 15 percent of the calories lost through your skin by convection. This means that air is circulating over your skin to move away the hot air envelope around you that has been formed by conduction, and replaces it with cooler air. The air movement aids elimination of calories of heat. A fan can help you feel cooler by speeding up the process. That is also why a wind makes you feel colder, and why the wind-chill reading is lower than the actual temperature readings.

The third important mechanism of eliminating heat is by evaporation. This is the same thing that happens with an evaporative cooler. You may not be aware of the fact that your skin perspires constantly. Since you are not aware of it, this is called insensible perspiration. It takes 0.56 calories to convert 1 ml of water to vapor. At ordinary room temperature, the moisture vaporized and lost from the surface of your skin, plus that from your lungs, accounts for about 17 calories per hr, or about 25 percent of the calories lost by your body at rest. About one-third of the heat lost by evaporation is lost through the lungs, and the other two-thirds from insensible perspiration from your skin.

Humidity has a major effect on how efficient your skin is in eliminating calories. As the humidity increases, the skin loses its ability to cool by evaporation. That is why sports and work in a combination of heat and humidity can be dangerous. When the humidity is high, the body has to depend mostly on radiation and convection to eliminate calories.

A relatively small amount, 5 percent, of calories of heat are lost through the heat in the urine and feces, and in warming the air inhaled into your lungs. These figures for heat-loss apply to a male who is moderately active, and is in caloric balance by exchanging 3,000 calories a day. They mean that 85 percent of the calories his body eliminates are eliminated through the skin. That should give you a new respect for the skin as an important factor in determining your calorie balance.

Your Circulation Is the Key

How efficient your skin is in eliminating calories, or in conserving them, depends on the blood flow through it. Your skin is a very vascular organ. It is filled with arteries, capillaries and veins. Its blood supply is far greater than would be needed to simply provide oxygen to the skin, or to provide nutrients. The main purpose of this large vascular supply is to enable your skin to function as a means of controlling elimination of calories, and thereby controlling your body temperature. Just by changing the amount of blood flow through the skin, its temperature can be changed from 15°C (59°F) to 38 ° (100.4°F). At a room temperature of 34°C (93.2°F), about 12 percent of the blood pumped by the heart goes to the skin. Certain parts of your body are able to have wide fluctuations in blood flow. The fingers are a good example. The blood flow through the fingers, when they are exposed to heat, may be 80 to 90 times their blood flow when they are exposed to cold.

The blood vessels in your skin are controlled by the sympathetic nerve fibers. That means their connections are through your spinal cord and to your hypothalamus. The hypothalamus, which has so much to do with ingesting calories and releasing calories through metabolism, also controls how your skin functions to eliminate calories. By increasing the blood flow through your skin, it facilitates the loss of calories of heat by radiation and convection.

Sweat Glands Help

Your eccrine sweat glands are a key part of evaporative cooling. You have two kinds of sweat glands, the apocrine and eccrine glands. The apocrine glands are really sex glands and provide secretions that cause odors. In the animal world the odors are sexually attractive. The eccrine glands produce sweat, which is mostly dilute salt water. There are about 2.5 million eccrine glands in your skin. In adults, they are most numerous in the sole of the foot and least numerous over the back. They are also numerous over the palms of the hands. They are chiefly controlled by the hypothalamus through the sympathic nerve fibers. Sometimes a person's nervous system is overactive and causes undesirable excessive sweating. I receive many letters like this one from people with this problem.

> DEAR DR. LAMB: I have had a very special problem as long as I can remember. It is profuse sweating of my hands and feet, 24 hours a day. This makes life very uncomfortable. During cold weather it makes my hands and feet become extremely cold. It prohibits handling of books and papers and other delicate items. It restricts my social life to a minimum.
>
> I'm now 26 years old and this problem seems to be getting worse as I get older. Now my armpits perspire profusely when I get excited. Tests to determine my problem show that my thyroid and other endocrine glands are normal. Is there any cure?

Having such overactive sweat glands is not a simple problem. Notice that the areas involved are the palms of the hands and soles of the feet. That is where the sweat glands are the most numerous. However, the nervous system can turn on the sweating mechanism of other areas, without causing excessive sweating of the hands and feet. The role of emotions in causing sweaty hands is a good example of how the brain controls the cooling mechanism. Also note that when she gets excited she begins to sweat under her arms. Here again is an area of abundant sweat glands and here, too, emotions affect their function through her brain.

Good evidence of the connection of the nerve tracts to the sweat glands is demonstrated by one means of controlling excessive sweating of the hands as told by this lady.

> DEAR DR. LAMB: My heart goes out to the lady with excessive sweating. I had the same problem. Mine was mainly my hands. No one can imagine how bad it really is. I never wanted to hold or shake anyone's hand, have change counted back into my hand or even sign my name in front of someone for fear the paper would be soaked.
>
> None of the medicines or preparations prescribed helped. Then I came across a neurosurgeon and underwent the surgical procedure at the age of 22. I have excellent results. Of course it was not inexpensive surgery, but for the difference it makes in your life, it's worth it.

The surgery the lady is talking about is severing the sympathetic nerve fibers that go to the palms of the hands. This makes it impossible for the brain to stimulate sweating of the palms. Another approach to the problem is to inactivate the sweat glands. In the case of underarm sweating, surgical removal of the portion of skin that contains the glands is sometimes done. There is now an electrical device called Drionic which consists of wet electrical pads that can be placed against the sweaty area and the current inactivates the sweat glands.

The role of sweating in lowering the body temperature is also seen in people who have night sweats. This lady's letter is an example:

DEAR DR. LAMB: I broke a hip eight months ago. I am doing very well, but I have had several periods of night sweats. They last from a few nights to weeks. I've had this last episode for three months now. They wake me up about 2:00 a.m. I have to change sheets and nightgown. By morning I am wet again.

Since the body temperature falls during the night, reaching its lowest point in the early morning hours, the body must eliminate heat. When there is a lot of heat to eliminate, the sweating mechanism is turned on and night sweats occur. This may be normal in some people. In others it is caused by some disease that results in increasing calorie release. It causes the body to use extra measures to try to eliminate extra calories. Since eating increases the release of calories of heat, one measure that helps in some people is to avoid large late meals. In such cases a light early meal is less likely to cause heat production during the night and turn on the sweating mechanism.

The role of the hypothalamus in controlling sweating may also be influenced by activity. An example is the increase in sweating that occurs at the beginning of exertion. This can occur before there has been any significant rise in body temperature, and is believed to occur from impulses from the brain's cortex.

As the environmental temperature increases, your body has to rely more and more on evaporative cooling to eliminate calories of heat. At temperatures above 35°C (95°F), evaporation accounts for nearly all the heat lost by your body. At an environmental temperature of 38°C (100.4°F), your body actually begins to gain heat by radiation from its surroundings. Eventually, the necessity to induce evaporative cooling is so overwhelming that sweat pours off the body. Unfortunately, that free-flowing sweat does not help cool your body much. It serves only to dehydrate the body. The real, effective evaporative cooling is from less obvious sweating before you get to the dripping stage.

The Skin's Temperature Sensors

Your skin is covered with temperature sensors. Some of these detect heat and others detect cold. These sensors relay signals through the sympathetic nerve fibers to your hypothalamus. They provide the main way your body senses external temperature. When you touch something cold, the appropriate sensors relay the cold signal. When you touch something hot, the hot sensors relay the hot signal. The skin temperature is really responsible for your sensation of being hot or cold. Of course, your skin temperature will be affected by the flow of hot blood through it, or the lack of it, and the effects of evaporative cooling.

There is a dual control mechanism between your hypothalamus and your skin that affects the heat production from the metabolic furnace and your heat loss through your skin. When the temperature of your hypothalamus exceeds 37°C (98.6°F), and at the same time the skin temperature rises, you will sweat. But if the temperature of your hypothalamus is below that level, your sweating mechanism is shut off, even if your skin temperature rises. Your hypothalamus senses your internal body temperature and has the ability to override heat loss through your skin to maintain the desired internal body temperature.

Evaporative cooling is also limited if your skin temperature is too cold. Sweating stops at skin temperatures below 29°C (84.2°F). Your body literally senses that you are losing heat, or will lose heat, and shuts down as much of the heat-loss mechanism as it can. Conversely, if your skin senses that you are getting too hot, the signal to the brain inhibits heat production by your body.

Heat loss through your skin is not just a passive mechanism that is turned on when your body gets too hot. You can lose calories through the skin because of cold exposure. As the calories are lost through radiation and convection, the body temperature will fall. With both the temperature in the hypothalamus dropping, and the skin temperature below normal, the body must turn on the metabolic furnace. It is a little like having left the air conditioner on full blast until the room temperature falls too low, which then turns on the furnace to raise the room temperature back to normal. The initial response is to release adrenaline. This boosts your cell metabolism and helps to fire your furnace to maintain your body temperature. Very little has been done to see how the calorie-loss mechanism through the skin can be used to advantage in eliminating unwanted calories of fat. But, when you want to lose fat, clearly, it is just as important to lose calories as it is to limit calorie intake.

Feeling Cold

How many times have you heard someone complain about being cold, while others in the same environment are comfortable, or actually warm? Or you may be one of these people who seem to feel the cold more than others. The explanation is in what is happening in the skin. This lady described the typical situation:

> DEAR DR. LAMB: I have a problem and no one seems to know what to do about it. I'm always cold. My husband sits in the same room with me in a short-sleeved shirt and is comfortable. I'm sitting there wearing a sweater and my heaviest clothes and I'm still cold. That is true even if the room temperature is in the high 70's. I need to keep the house warm to be comfortable and my husband complains because the house is too hot. I've had tests done and my thyroid is all right and the doctors don't find anything wrong with me.
>
> I'm a little overweight. I weigh 156 pounds and am 5 feet 4 inches tall. I'm 58 years old. Do you have any idea what the problem is? My husband is 59 and he is rather thin. I thought thin people didn't tolerate cold as well as overweight people.

When the blood flow to your skin is limited, you will feel cold. Those nerve fibers in your skin are not being warmed. At the same time, because there is decreased heat loss from your skin, your internal body temperature may be quite normal. When you take your temperature, you may be surprised to find that it is in the normal range. Conversely, when a person feels hot and thinks he may have a fever, he may find his body temperature is actually normal. That individual is eliminating heat through the skin, and has an increased blood flow through the skin, which is effectively cooling his internal temperature to normal levels.

The overweight person who feels cold is of special interest because she is decreasing her loss of calories through the skin and that means her body is using fewer calories, even if her thyroid and other endocrine glands are perfectly normal. Her brain is trying to keep her from losing calories and trying to maintain her level of body fat, even though she may have more body fat stores than she wants.

This lady's husband is thin. He is losing calories through his skin and feels comfortable. The calorie loss through his skin indicates that the brain is trying to eliminate calories and keep him at his present weight on the thin side.

One of the most effective things a person can do to eliminate that feeling of being cold is to exercise. Physical activity turns on the metabolic furnace and releases heat. At the same time it turns on the skin's heat-loss mechanism and a person feels warmer. You can notice this when you go out in the cold. At first you feel uncomfortable, but as you exercise you begin to feel warm and the cold no longer bothers you.

The extreme of the problem in the difference between feeling hot or cold and the actual internal body temperature is often noted in relation to a fever. During the time that the body is accumulating heat to raise the body temperature level, the heat-loss mechanism in the skin may be slowed. You may not feel hot or may actually feel chilly, but when you take your temperature, it is elevated. As the febrile illness peaks, you may feel hot and begin to sweat. When you take your temperature, it is falling. You feel hot because your body is cooling. This sudden break in a fever, signaled by turning on the heat-loss mechanism and sweating, gives rise to the old observation that when a person has had a fever and starts to sweat, he is getting better. The crisis is over. All of this explains why feeling hot or cold is not a very good indicator of what your internal body temperature really is.

Cold Exposure

While heat loss by evaporative cooling increases as the environmental temperature rises, the opposite occurs as environmental temperature falls. As the environmental temperature falls below 28°C (82.4°F), the heat loss by radiation and convection increases, while loss by evaporation decreases. If you were sitting nude in a temperature of 23°C (73.4°F), you would be very uncomfortable and start shivering. This has been called the critical temperature. Shivering is a natural form of heat production. Even before shivering begins, muscle tension rises, and that causes the release of heat. Shivering increases heat production by the muscles. It can triple the heat production above its resting level and raise the body temperature. The role of muscles in this action has been proved by paralyzing the muscles in animals with drugs which stop this compensatory mechanism against decreasing body temperature.

There is ample evidence that your brain controls your body temperature. If one area of the hypothalamus is damaged, the body temperature may soar. This is an especially dreaded complication of brain surgery. The rise in temperature is an emergency and can result in death. Measures such as packing the body in ice and using cold water enemas are employed to try to control the body temperature. Some medicines, including the barbiturates, seem to be helpful in turning off the excessive heat production. In contrast, if another area of the hypothalamus is damaged, body temperature falls to dangerously low levels and must be maintained by artificial means. A unique experiment that demonstrated the hypothalamus' role in eliminating heat was to heat a cat's hypothalamus with diathermy, a form of radio waves that causes deep heating. This caused the cat to pant and its paws to sweat.

The importance of heat loss in terms of body weight is well known to every farmer who must feed livestock in cold weather. When livestock are exposed to cold weather, it is essential to increase their calorie intake, or they lose weight. That is why feed-lot operators hate cold weather. The increased feed bills decrease or wipe out their profits. A warm barn to provide shelter for animals significantly cuts down on the feed bills. The same thing happens to people exposed to cold.

Studies have shown that cold may double the resting calorie requirements. In polar expeditions, the men involved in sledging operations for eight to ten hours daily used 5,000 to 6,500 calories a day and still lost weight. This is well in excess of the calories a man can use while involved in maximum physical effort for eight hours a day in temperate climate. Men who traveled by motorized toboggans in the Antarctic, between October and December, lost between 4.4 and 9.2 kilograms (9.7 to 20.2 pounds) and used an average of 3,500 calories a day.

Survival, when exposed to cold temperature, often depends on how effective your body is at conserving heat. If you lose calories rapidly, you have less chance for survival. That is the real basis for some of the survival instructions. High on the list is not to drink alcohol. When a person drinks alcohol, he may *feel* warmer. The alcohol causes the blood flow through the skin to increase and the skin feels warmer. It is the alcoholic flush that you see in a person who drinks that does this.

The increased flow of hot blood that raises the skin temperature in a person with normal internal body temperature (37°C, 98.6°F) induces the "whiskey sweats." In the cold, increased circulation will speed up the loss of calories and speed up the depletion of the body energy stores. An individual who drinks is apt to reach a critical low body temperature much earlier, and die from cold exposure. It is no accident that many of the hypothermia victims picked up in alleys in cold months have been drinking alcohol.

While exercise is great for health, it is bad for cold survival. If you are not in a survival situation, it helps you feel warm and is no threat to your health, but *if you are isolated in the cold and trying to survive, exercise can kill you.* Turning on the heat-loss mechanism through exercise increases the blood flow through your skin and makes you feel warm, but you are literally exhausting your body's energy stores. When they are exhausted, hypothermia and death will follow.

Survival time in cold water is very limited. There is a rapid loss of body heat through conduction. Water is 25 times as conductive of heat as air. As a result, there is a rapid transfer of calories through the skin to the water. As you might expect from the foregoing comments, individuals who tend to be fat have a much longer survival time in cold water than skinny people.

Summary 4

1. The law of conservation of energy means:
    Calories consumed − calories used = calories stored as body fat.
2. You are constantly losing calories through your skin—day and night.

3. You lose heat through your skin by radiation, conduction, convection and evaporation.
4. About 85 percent of the calories lost from the body are eliminated through the skin.
5. Your brain controls blood flow through your skin. The blood flow affects how fast you lose calories, and how many.
6. The brain controls sweating and evaporative cooling.
7. Feeling hot or cold is not a good indicator of your internal body temperature. When you feel cold, the skin is conserving calories. When you feel hot, the skin is eliminating calories.
8. Exposure to cold increases calorie loss through the skin.
9. Drinking alcoholic beverages increases calorie loss through the skin and decreases survival time during cold exposure.
10. Exercise in cold survival increases calorie loss and shortens survival time.
11. Exposure to cold water speeds up loss of calories through the skin.

Chapter 5

Your Calorie Balance

Now, you have seen how your brain controls the "calories in" and the "calories out." When you are in caloric balance, the "calories in" equal the "calories out." If you are in positive calorie balance, your body will store the calories it does not eliminate. Those stored calories are body fat. Since the brain controls the calories in and the calories out, obviously it must control the stored calories or your body fat, at least indirectly. The brain also has an effect on where those fat stores of calories are put. When you are in negative calorie balance, your body is eliminating more calories than you are consuming, and your body has to provide the difference. If you are on a sensible diet program, that difference in calories will come from the calories stored as body fat. If not, they will come from glycogen stored from carbohydrate, or your body protein. But before we explore these ramifications, let's take another look at how your brain, nerves and endocrine glands work together to control your calorie balance.

Your Brain's Automatic Nerve Control

There are three main systems involved with the brain in maintaining your calorie balance. The first is your hypothalamus-sympathetic nervous system. Your hypothalamus, in the floor of your brain, connects to nerve tracts that pass down the brain into your spinal cord. At each vertebral level, nerve fibers exit from your spinal cord and form a chain of nerves, called the sympathetic nerves. Nerves from this system go to your entire body. You do not have any control over these nerves. They are automatic, and part of the autonomic nervous system. Sometimes, the autonomic nervous system is called the involuntary nervous system.

For the most part, the sympathetic nerve fibers work by using norepinephrine (noradrenaline), and some use epinephrine (adrenaline). These chemicals are essential to transmit the impulses that pass down these nerves. Some of the fibers do use another chemical, acetylcholine, to transmit impulses. The sympathetic nerve fibers even connect to the center of your adrenal gland, where large quantities of epinephrine and a small amount of norepinephrine are formed. These hormones are liberated when you are under stress. Sympathetic nerve stimulation, and the release of adrenaline, will increase your metabolism, immediately releasing heat inside the body. Adrenaline release is one of the first measures your body can take to protect itself when you are exposed to cold. This is a temporary measure.

In addition, the sympathetic nerves can control how heat is eliminated through your skin. They do this through the control of blood flow through your skin, which affects radiation and convection, as well as through control of eccrine sweat glands that affect evaporative cooling. By varying both circulation and sweating, the skin can either conserve calories of heat or eliminate calories of heat. It is worth noting that information from the skin sensors, regarding whether you are hot or cold, is transmitted through the sympathetic nerve fibers back to the hypothalamus.

The epinephrine and norepinephrine sympathetic nervous system, related to your hypothalamus, has its counterpart in the parasympathetic nervous system. This is the second mechanism the brain has to control your calorie balance. It is the other main part of the autonomic nervous system. In terms of calorie balance, this is the vagus nerve. It originates directly from the brain stem that connects to the spinal cord. Since your vagus nerve originates directly from the brain, it is called a cranial nerve. It sends fibers to most of your internal organs, including the heart, lungs and abdominal viscera. It transmits impulses by using the chemical acetylcholine. In a way, you can think of the parasympathetic nervous system and the sympathetic nervous system as the "yin and yang" or the positive and negative, or the north and south. They tend to have opposite functions in the body. The sympathetic nerves speed up your heart, and the vagus nerve from the parasympathetic system slows down your heart.

The vagus nerve fibers stimulate the islets of Langerhans in the pancreas. In this way, they cause the secretion of insulin. That is important in enabling glucose to enter the cells, so it can be burned to carbon dioxide and water to release energy. The insulin is also important in formation of fat for storage of calories, and inhibits the mobilization of fat from fat cells.

Fibers from the vagus nerve connect with the stretch receptors in your stomach, and tell your brain when your stomach is full. They also provide sensors to the rest of the digestive system and send back additional information to the brain on whether or not you need to eat more.

Your Brain Controls Hormones

The third calorie-balance system affected by your brain is the neuroendocrine axis. Your endocrine glands do not simply function on their own. Most of those associated with calorie control are affected by your pituitary gland, located just under your brain. This master gland is anatomically connected by a stalk to the floor of the hypothalamus. Perhaps more importantly, it is affected by nerve fibers from the brain and by brain chemicals. The pituitary releases a hormone, called the thyrotropic hormone, that stimulates the thyroid gland. If you didn't have a pituitary gland, or it didn't release this hormone, your thyroid gland would not function properly. The absence of normal thyroid function would decrease your body's ability to metabolize foodstuffs adequately, and your metabolic furnace would literally quit putting out the necessary heat.

Another hormone from the pituitary stimulates the adrenal cortex, which surrounds the adrenal center that produces epinephrine and norepinephrine. This cortex area is the source of the corticosteroid hormones, and they also affect metabolism.

Still other pituitary hormones stimulate the sex glands (gonads), the ovaries in females and the testicles in males. These hormones control the menstrual cycle in females and also the sexual cycle in males. By stimulating the development and function of the ovaries, the pituitary indirectly causes the development of normal body-fat deposits characteristic of the female. And by stimulating the action of the testicles, they cause the muscular and bone development characteristic of the male.

The role of the pituitary gland doesn't stop there. It also forms growth hormone. Your pituitary gland's release of growth hormone is also under the control of the brain. As the name implies, this hormone stimulates tissue growth, which requires calories of energy and is part of your energy balance system. It also diminishes fat deposits while stimulating growth.

These three systems of the brain are all integrated and are influenced by other centers of the brain. The higher functions of the brain have a greater input and control of events in humans than in animals. We can literally use our cerebral cortex, and the knowledge we have learned, to manipulate our response to stimuli provoked by the energy balance system. That means you can refuse to eat foods that are high in calories, or you can force yourself to exercise. Your energy balance system is influenced by inputs from your eyes, nose, taste buds and a thousand other cues. Your cortex may control your physical activity, and the effects are relayed into your energy balance system. Your hypothalamus also contains your thermostat. It perceives from the blood what your internal body temperature is. It literally controls your energy balance system to maintain your body temperature at the desired level. Your brain is very complex. The details of how it performs all these functions have not been fully established, but what your brain "does" is rather clear, even if the "how" is not entirely understood.

Winners and Losers

With a basic concept of how your body eliminates calories, not just how many calories you consume, you can begin to understand some of the mysteries of the weighting game. Let's take the problem of the two ladies who both weighed 180 pounds and were similar in lifestyle, health, diet and exercise. One loses body fat and the other does not, even though both are consuming the same number of calories. Think of your simple energy equation: Energy in − Energy out = Energy stored. If one woman is losing fat, which means she is in negative calorie balance, she must be eliminating more calories of heat than calories consumed. The other lady, consuming the same number of calories, must not be losing as many calories of heat. Why, is less clear, but the problem is related to heat exchange. You have to make this conclusion to conform to the laws of the conservation of energy. The lady losing fat has not found a magical way to destroy calories, and the lady who is not losing fat has not found a magical way to create calories. Remember that energy is neither created nor destroyed, or, stated another way, calories are neither created nor destroyed. But your body can process calories in different ways, and those different ways can affect whether or not you lose body fat when you are on a diet and exercise program.

Forming Body Fat

When you are in positive caloric balance, your body forms fat. Your body can also produce and store glycogen, which is a starch formed by connecting glucose molecules together. Approximately 70 grams of glycogen is stored in the liver. This glycogen is readily available to be converted to glucose and used to maintain the blood glucose level. There are about 200 grams of glycogen stored in the skeletal muscles. But this glycogen cannot be removed, and is used only for the energy requirements of the muscles. As a result, the number of calories that can be stored as glycogen is rather limited. There is also a pool of amino acids from protein in your body fluids and tissues that is available to use to build new structures and chemicals, such as enzymes. The amount of amino acids that can be stored is limited, too. As a result, any extra calories must be used either for growth, which stops in most people when they are mature, or stored as body fat. Your body can use amino acids from excess protein intake and glucose from carbohydrates to form fat. In humans, most of the fat is formed in the liver, then released as triglycerides (fat) into the blood. Your blood carries it to fat cells, where it is deposited.

Your white fat cells are really storage tanks. They can expand to accommodate the amount of fat that needs to be stored. They do not break down the fat, or release energy. The fat stores in the cells do turn over rapidly. The fat that was stored two days ago may be mobilized and hauled off by your circulation to other cells to be burned to release energy, while new fat is being stored. The fat you store doesn't just stay there. It is constantly turning over.

If you study the complex chemical changes involved in converting carbohydrate to fat, you will find something very interesting. It doesn't require oxygen to form fatty acids. That is because the fatty acids are essentially free of oxygen. It doesn't require any oxygen to convert amino acids from protein to fatty acids either, for the same reason. When you consume excess calories in the form of carbohydrates or protein, they are quickly converted to fat. Oxygen is only used to burn foods, carbohydrates, proteins or fats, to release energy. When you consume extra calories, and the excess calories of energy are stored as fat, this will not generate any body heat or require any oxygen. The body heat produced, and the oxygen used, is only related to the calories used, not those that are stored.

You probably think of insulin in relation to diabetes, but it has an important role in storing calories as body fat. The formation of fatty acids is facilitated by insulin. It follows that not only will low insulin levels decrease your body's ability to utilize glucose, but a lack of insulin will inhibit the conversion of excess carbohydrates, or amino acids, to fat. In the advanced diabetic, this can contribute to the weight loss that occurs. The insulin dependent diabetic has trouble forming fat.

Fat is really a chemical combination of fatty acids and glycerol, the same glycerine used in hand lotion. That combination of fatty acids and glycerol, called glyceride, is what you see when you look at the fat on the meat you buy at the market. It is also what is in the fat under the skin. When three fatty acids are combined with glycerol to form glyceride it is called a triglyceride. When you hear the term "triglyceride," just think fat.

To get fat out of storage in your fat cells, the combination between glycerol and fatty acids has to be broken apart, a process called lipolysis. Then the free fatty acid can be hauled away to other cells to be burned to release energy. Insulin inhibits lipolysis, thus making it difficult for your body to mobilize fat deposits. In that case, your body has to search for energy stores other than stored fat. That is one reason why people who have increased amounts of insulin, as in hypoglycemia, may get fat. They need energy, and must eat to provide it, because they can't get the fat back out of their fat cells. Insulin both promotes fat formation and storage of fat. In contrast, epinephrine (adrenaline) facilitates lipolysis and the mobilization of fat.

What Kind of Fat Cells?

There are small fat cells and large fat cells. Whether a person is overweight or not depends upon the total amount of fat in all cells. But there is a very important point, which is still being studied, that can influence a person's lifelong tendency to be overweight. It is the number of fat cells that are formed. Once you are an adult, the number of fat cells you have remains constant, unless a surgeon cuts them out. Even with the most stringent diet, the number remains the same. As a person gets thin, the fat cells just get smaller, but do not disappear. There is some evidence that the more fat cells you have, the more likely you are to have a problem with weight control.

There are two periods in life when a person is most likely to increase the number of fat cells. The first period is within the first two years of life. The second is around the time of puberty. This suggests that it may not be prudent to overfeed your child, and have a fat baby. It also suggests that teen-agers should avoid getting fat. That is not a recommendation for being too thin, either. Once puberty is over, you may be set for life with your fat cells.

During the time of fat cell multiplication, the size of the fat cells may be important. When the fat cell reaches a critical size, it may duplicate itself to form more fat cells. In the main, it seems that it is easier for a person with fewer fat cells to lose body fat and keep it off. The most typical adult-onset type of obesity doesn't involve an increased number of fat cells. The fat cells are simply quite large.

Dr. Jules Hirsch of Rockefeller University originally proposed the idea of fat cell multiplication in early life about 20 years ago. Originally, he suggested that overfeeding the baby might predispose to more fat cells and predispose to adult obesity. Most of this work was done in animals as it is difficult or impossible to do similar studies in infants. Today he believes that both enlarged fat cells and increased numbers of fat cells may be important—the person with average obesity having enlarged fat cells and the very obese person having both an increased number of fat cells and enlarged fat cells.

Dr. Douglas S. Lewis of the Southwest Foundation for Biomedical Research in San Antonio, Texas, used baboons as a model to study feeding habits and subsequent obesity. Baboons are similar to humans in terms of body fat patterns. He observed that female baboons that were overfed from birth to 4 months of age gained excess amounts of fat at the onset of puberty. This was not observed in male baboons, which suggests a hormonal factor. Puberty in the female does trigger increased body fat deposits.

Catabolic or Anabolic

Up to this point, in discussing how your body processes calories, I have used the term metabolism. But that is a general term which refers to the chemical changes that occur when your foodstuffs are processed. Metabolism really consists of two types of actions. One is the breakdown of substances, which is called "catabolism." That is what happens when your tissues are breaking down and you are losing weight, or foodstuffs are broken down to release energy for your body. The other phase is the building phase, with the formation of new structures or chemicals. That is called "anabolism."

The breakdown and release of energy as calories of heat is the catabolic process, but the formation and storage of fat is an anabolic process. So is the formation of enzymes or other important body chemicals, or the formation of new tissue, as required for growth. The anabolic process requires energy. When amino acids are hooked together to form new proteins for muscle, that requires energy. When a young person is in the growing phase, he needs to be in positive calorie balance, and is storing calories in the new structures he is forming in the anabolic process. As long as the calories are used for growing muscle and body structures, you can watch him consume lots of calories and not get fat. The same is true when you develop muscles through exercise. The anabolic process does not use oxygen or generate heat, but is a calorie storage process. The catabolic process uses oxygen to burn substances and does release heat. When muscles, or other essential body structures, are catabolized for energy, then the process requires oxygen, generates heat and releases calories. That also means our basic equation for calorie balance needs to be slightly modified to:

Calories in − calories used = calories deposited as fat + calories used in growth.

Note this remains consistent with the law of conservation of energy.

Putting It All Together

Let us now look at a new diagram that explains very simply how your calorie balance works. Your brain controls your "calories in" as foodstuffs. It also controls your "calories out" through heat loss, pri-

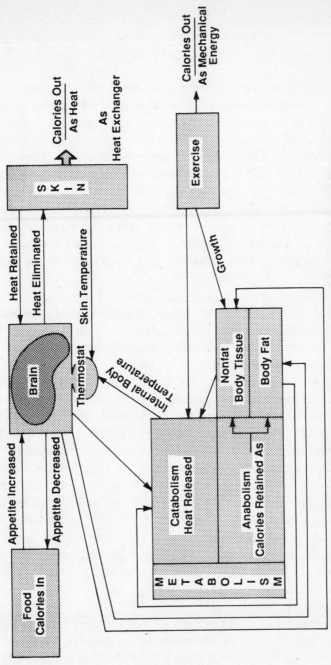

The brain receives signals from all functions that are related to calorie balance, controlling calories in and calories out.

marily through your skin. Your brain will control these two functions in relation to your body temperature, sensed by the thermostat in your hypothalamus, and from your skin temperature relayed to the hypothalamus.

As your foodstuffs are catabolized, they will release the calories of heat they contained when you consumed them—4 calories per gram of carbohydrate or protein, and 9 calories per gram of fat. If they are not to be used, they are converted to body fat, an anabolic process. Later, your fat stores can be mobilized and catabolized to release heat. Or, the calories not used for heat may be used for growth of body tissues, or the formation of needed chemical compounds such as enzymes or some hormones. The calories released by catabolism, whether from your food or your fat stores or tissue, will cause your body temperature to rise, and that will be sensed by your brain's thermostat. Then your brain will simply increase the calories of heat released from your skin.

If you lose heat from your skin, and need more heat to maintain your body temperature, your brain can increase your appetite to provide more calories from your foodstuffs, or your body can mobilize fat. If neither of these are readily available, body protein and stored glycogen can be catabolized.

Where does exercise fit into this scheme of things? It stimulates catabolism to release energy. Less than 25 percent of the energy released during exercise is used for mechanical energy. The rest, over 75 percent, is released as heat. Depending on the type of activity, and your physiological state, exercise may also increase muscle growth, an anabolic process, and use calories in the anabolic process. So exercise can stimulate a healthy growth of tissue and use energy that way, or it can stimulate catabolism, releasing heat. As such, it drives the heat-loss mechanism through your brain. From a calorie-balance point of view, exercise is an attractive and healthy way to turn on your heat-loss mechanism and control your calorie balance, rather than deprive your body of foodstuffs that contain important nutrients. *Limiting your calorie intake shuts down your energy system. Exercise stimulates your energy system.* It is really that simple.

It is important to learn to think of calorie balance, not just pounds. *You can actually gain weight and be losing calories.* The healthy way that occurs is by developing muscles while you are mobilizing and eliminating body fat. The basis for this is in the number of calories in lean muscle as opposed to body fat. A pound of lean muscle (454 grams) contains only about 600 calories. One reason for that is because over 70 percent of its weight is water. An average figure for the calories in a pound of body fat is 3,500 calories. Only about 15 percent of its weight is water. If you exercise, and limit your calories at the same time, so that you develop a pound of muscle while you lose a pound of body fat, you will weigh the same. But you will have lost 2,900 calories (3,500 - 600). Even if you gained five pounds of muscle, while you lost one pound of fat, you would still have lost about 500 calories despite gaining four pounds of weight. Usually, it is not a good idea to lose protein tissue such as muscle. It is often healthy to develop additional muscle. For most people, the goal should be to eliminate excess unhealthy body fat, while maintaining or developing muscles.

Summary 5

1. Stress activates your sympathetic nervous system and adrenal glands to release adrenaline—your stress hormone. This increases the release of calories.
2. Your vagus nerve stimulates the release of insulin.
3. Insulin promotes the movement of glucose into the cells where it can be oxidized to release calories of energy.
4. Insulin is essential to the formation of fat to store energy.
5. The brain controls your pituitary gland. Your pituitary gland controls your thyroid. The amount of thyroid hormone you produce affects metabolism to release calories in your cells.
6. Your pituitary gland stimulates your adrenal cortex to release corticosteroid hormones which affect your cell metabolism.
7. The brain controls your pituitary gland's ability to stimulate the sex glands. The sex hormones influence the development of fat stores.
8. Your brain controls your pituitary gland's release of growth hormone which promotes growth and diminishes fat deposits.
9. The calories from an excess intake of both carbohydrates and protein are converted to fat and stored.
10. It doesn't require oxygen to form body fat from excess calorie intake. Forming body fat does not produce any calories of heat.
11. Insulin inhibits the mobilization of body fat to be used for energy.

This, plus the action of insulin to form fat, is why people who have hypoglycemia from excess insulin tend to have excess fat stores.

12. Excessive calorie intake in infancy and at puberty may increase the number of fat cells, the tendency to have large fat cells or both. This may contribute to adult obesity.

13. Forming body proteins and growth require energy to hook the amino acids and other chemicals together. That is why a high calorie intake during growth may not cause obesity.

14. Exercise turns on your metabolic furnace and drives your energy system.

15. Limiting calorie intake shuts down your energy system.

16. You can gain weight while losing calories. That happens when you increase your muscle size while losing body fat.

Chapter 6

What Should You Weigh?

There is a big difference between needing to lose weight and wanting to lose weight. There are valid health reasons for many people to shed excess pounds of body fat, but many people playing the weighting game have no reason to lose weight at all, in terms of health. A lot of these people may actually be harming their health by being overzealous in staying thin. The most common motivation for people to want to lose weight is to improve their appearance. There is nothing wrong with that, if you are honest with yourself, and recognize that is why you are doing it. But you must be careful not to overdo it to the point of damaging your health. I'll discuss the problem of undernutrition later. Many people have a complete misconception about what they should weigh. Indeed, even the experts have had problems because they try to make rules that fit everyone. Determining what you should weigh is one of those areas where you should follow the rule, "individualize, don't generalize."

Lessons from Nature

We were all born with many predetermined factors that will affect our lives. People do tend to stay at the same level of fatness, despite wide variations in the number of calories consumed and their level of exercise. The same thing is observed in the animal kingdom. If you leave animals alone, and give them unlimited access to the foods they would eat in a natural setting, they will stay at about the same body weight. There are some animals that have inherited characteristics to

63

become obese. That has been amply demonstrated in the laboratory. Certain strains of mice are prone to get fat, and are used in the laboratory because of that inherited characteristic. Ordinary rats will not get fat on their natural foods. When they eat more than they should, their brown fat simply increases heat production, and the excess calories are eliminated as heat. But the Zucker rat has a genetic defect that prevents it from being able to respond in this manner to excess calories. As a result, the Zucker rats get fat. That doesn't mean you can't make the ordinary laboratory rat fat. You can do this by substituting high-calorie foods for his usual foods. Evidently, the rat is unable to distinguish between calorie-rich foods and those that are not. As the rat continues to eat the same amount, it consumes far more calories than its "calories out" mechanism can handle, and it gets fat. There is an important lesson here about body fat. You can inherit factors that predispose you to being overweight, or you can get fat by following poor dietary habits. Some people have both problems.

Every farmer concerned with raising livestock knows the importance of blood lines, or genes. Some cattle are beef cattle and tend to be fat. A good beef animal will grow rapidly, and put on weight easily, while consuming a limited amount of food. Indeed, cattlemen have breed animals to do just that. In contrast, a dairy cow may be rather lean, but she will produce lots of milk. She literally uses her nutrition to produce milk, not fat deposits. Dairy cows have been bred with special characteristics to do just this. You can affect how fat the beef animal will be by how you feed him, and you can affect how much milk the dairy cow will produce by how you feed her, but the basic genetic characteristics are unchanged. You will not be able to get the beef cow to produce the same amount of milk that the prize dairy cow will produce, and you will not get the dairy cow to "beef up" and get as fat as the beef cow. You can extend this principle to pigs and almost every animal species. It applies to chickens as well. Some breeds are developed to produce lots of eggs, others are bred to produce a lot of meat. Everywhere you look in the animal kingdom the message is clear. Genes do make a difference.

You don't need to stop with the animal kingdom. Look at the plant world. Plants have been developed to grow and thrive in relatively adverse environments. Some are designed to produce lots of seed. Others are designed to produce lots of foliage. Some trees are developed to grow rapidly but many have a short life-span, while others grow slowly and live for centuries. You cannot escape the genetic connection in nature, and it is unreasonable to think you would in humans.

You were born with a life script that determines what you should weigh, and how much fat you should have, at various stages of your life. It is a lot like inheriting factors that will determine how tall you will be. These characteristics can be influenced by what you do, but you often have to mistreat your body to change them. A case in point is what happened to the growth of Japanese children before and after World War II. Before the war, the children were small, as were their parents. Their diet was low in protein. After the war, as the diet improved, the children grew much faster, to the point that the furniture for classrooms no longer fit. In many countries where nutrition is not adequate today, the average child's growth is retarded and he may never reach his actual inherited potential. You also inherit characteristics that should keep you within a range of body fatness. But if you really "pig out" on high-calorie foods, or are too inactive, you can override those limits and become overweight in an unhealthy way.

Nature or Nurture

A tug of war has long existed between those who believe that we are primarily influenced by environment, versus those who believe we inherit characteristics as part of our genetic makeup that determine what we are. It is the old "nature or nurture" debate. This has extended to our understanding of being overweight. The genetic group has insisted that we inherit the characteristics to be overweight, normal or skinny. The environmentalists have insisted with equal fervor that it is all a matter of what eating habits are learned within the family environment. They have supported the idea that the reason being overweight seems to occur in families is because of learned habits within the family, while the genetic proponents have said family characteristics are evidence of the genetic connection. The typical situation that stimulates all this debate is described in this letter.

DEAR DR. LAMB: I am a 45-year-old female, 5 feet 2 and weigh 142 pounds. Naturally I'm trying to lose weight. It has always been a losing battle for me. Even when I diet, I don't seem to lose weight.

My sister tells me this is because our family tends to be overweight. She claims it is a family characteristic and there is nothing I can do about it. But I have lost weight in the past when I have really dieted. Of course, it took a lot of effort. And the worst part is that it came right back.

My sister says that the reason I gain it back so quickly is because I'm supposed to be heavy. I would like to know the truth. Can I lose weight by dieting and is being overweight inherited or caused by eating too many calories?

That long-running debate took a decided turn in favor of genes when a recent study of adopted children was published in the *New England Journal of Medicine*, January 23, 1986. Dr. Albert Stunkard and colleagues at the University of Pennsylvania; the Psykologisk, Institut, Kommunehospitalet in Copenhagen, Denmark, and the University of Health Sciences in Houston, Texas, found a way to test the nature or nurture concepts. In Denmark, there is a register of the natural parents of adopted children. This made it possible to identify people who had been adopted and study them in relation to both their genetic parents and their adoptive parents. The study included 540 adults who had been adopted. It involved classifying people into four groups of relative fatness: thin, median weight, overweight and obese. They also used height-weight measurements to assess the body-mass index.

The Danish study showed a clear-cut relationship between the body-mass index of the adopted subjects and their genetic parents. This was true in all four groups of thin, median weight, overweight and obese children and their genetic parents. There was no relationship between the body-mass index of the adopted subjects and their adoptive parents. This is strong evidence for a genetic influence on relative body fatness, as opposed to environmental influences. It is entirely consistent with what occurs in the animal and plant world. In short, humans are not that different from the rest of the creatures and plants of the world. If you are on the heavy side, you may have just cause to blame the tendency on your parents. At this point, you can even predict which children are apt to be overweight. About 80 percent of the children of two obese parents will also be obese, but only 14 percent of offspring from two parents of normal weight are apt to be obese.

Still another study by Stunkard and colleagues added more support to the genetic concept. They studied what happened to 1,974 male pairs of identical twins and 1,097 pairs of male non-identical twins. They were able to get the original records from men who entered military service. Then they studied them again 25 years later. They found that the identical twins were quite similar to each other at the time they entered military service and again 20 years later. The similarity in the identical twins was twice as great as in the non-identical twins. That is a much stronger relationship than you might think. Not only do identical twins have identical genes, but non-identical twins also inherit some of the same genes, just as two brothers who are not twins often do. Thus, the observation that patterns of obesity were twice as similar in identical twins compared to non-identical twins is quite significant. The other point is that you are looking at a span of 25 years, suggesting that the pattern of obesity at different stages of a person's life is indeed a life-script and is inherited.

You might think these observations are very discouraging in terms of losing weight. They are, to some extent. But they do not mean you can't influence that tendency to be overweight. Some of the ways this might be accomplished are evident from the fundamental relationships in your calorie balance system. It is important, though, to recognize that if you were designed to be the family automobile, it is rather futile to treat your chassis like the sleek new sports car on the block. *It is not smart to fight your body. The question that faces you then is, are you overweight when your body says you should not be, or are you only apparently overweight, since that is what your weight is supposed to be?*

Your Fat Cell Receptors

It is not just a question of how much body fat you have, but where it is. That, too, is probably an inherited characteristic.

How genes affect where the fat goes was studied by researchers from Laval University, Quebec, Canada, in six pairs of identical twins. They fed these young men 1,000 calories a day more than they needed. Their physical activity was limited, and their eating was monitored for 22 days. Each pair of twins tended to put fat on in the same places, showing that it is not just the amount of extra fat that is genetically predetermined but also where it goes.

There was an interesting sidelight to the data on these young men. Despite consuming 1,000 extra calories a day for 22 days, the average gain in body fat was only 1.1 kilogram, or 2.4 pounds. The 22,000 extra calories should have resulted in 6.3 pounds of body fat. Why didn't they gain as much body fat as might be expected from overeating? As I have pointed out, the body has a wonderful tendency to maintain your weight. The most likely explanation is that the metabolic furnace was turned up and more heat was eliminated. These men not only consumed more calories, but they also lost more calories. The net result was a much smaller gain in body fat than might have been expected.

Where body fat goes is certainly related to whether you are male or female. Men tend to develop excess fat over the abdomen, described by the undignified term of the "beer belly." Women tend to have fat deposits over the buttocks and thighs. This can make a person very unhappy, as this letter suggests.

> DEAR DR. LAMB: I am a 19-year-old female. I'm 5 feet 7 inches tall and weight 127 pounds. I don't consider myself fat, just out of shape. My rear end and back of my legs seem to blend together. I would like to know how to firm up these areas and get rid of fat.

For an unusual distribution of fat deposits, the Hottentots of Africa certainly are near the head of the list. They have an inherited characteristic to develop a very large fat deposit over the buttocks, like a large pillow over the gluteal region, as a distinctive characteristic. Moreover, it is difficult to eliminate the fat from these special regions. As almost everyone knows who has gone on a diet, you tend to lose weight in the face first, and lose that large abdomen or fat hips last. It is a cruel trick of nature that you lose fat last from the very places that you would like to lose fat the most. There is a reason for this.

Why does the fat distribution follow these patterns? It is related to the characteristics of the fat cells themselves. For a cell to be stimulated, it must have a receptor for the nerve action. This is a lot like saying that before you can plug in your TV set, there has to be an electrical receptor. Where that receptor is determines where your TV set is going to go. Fat cells have two types of receptors, called $alpha_2$ and beta receptors. Norepinephrine tends to stimulate the $alpha_2$ receptors, but may have some effect on the beta receptors as well. Epinephrine tends to have an equal effect on both the $alpha_2$

and beta receptors. The important point about these receptors and your fat cells is that the receptor determines whether fat is being stored in your fat cells, or being broken down and released. The beta receptors stimulate the fat cells to break down stored fat. The fat cells with these receptors are the ones that unload first, when your body needs to use fat. But the alpha$_2$ receptors cause the fat cells to resist the breakdown of fat and enhance fat storage. They tend to make fat cells enlarge.

Studies by Drs. Jules Hirsch, Rudolph Leibel and Irving Faust of Rockefeller University have demonstrated that individuals with a lot of fat over the abdomen have fat cells in that location which are rich in alpha$_2$ receptors, and people with fat deposits over the buttocks and thighs also have cells in those locations that are rich in alpha$_2$ receptors. The young lady probably has fat retaining cells over her buttocks and the back of her thighs.

Now you know why those "love handles" around your sides will not go away even though your face is sagging from weight loss. The location of those resistant fat cells with the alpha$_2$ receptors is the reason. The deposits with these receptors are most resistant to losing fat. No amount of abdominal exercises, twisting, heating, massaging or torturing the area is going to make these fat deposits disappear. *That is why spot reducing will not, and does not, work.* You cannot change the character of the fat cells' receptors with any of these procedures. About the only way you can get rid of those fat cells is to cut them out. That sounds drastic, but it is realistic. To make those fat cells give up their fat you would really need to achieve a state of near-starvation that would be a serious threat to your health.

Jules Hirsch and colleagues' studies also suggest that the number of fat cells may influence the brain to promote fat deposits. They have observed that the number of fat cells a person has tends to remain constant. In a study of rat littermates, they noted that all the rats tended to develop the same degree of fatness while on the same diet. They surgically removed half of the fat cells from some of the littermates. After that, they were just about half as fat as their normal littermates. These investigators believe that the number of fat cells you have is an important factor in determining how fat you will be. Moreover, where those fat cells are located, and what kind of receptors they have, will determine the distribution of your fat deposits.

Do these findings observed in rats apply to humans? Yes. According to Leibel, people who were obese and reduced their body weight still had three times as many fat cells as people who were never overweight. The fat cells were small after losing weight, but numerous.

What about cellulite? The idea that individuals with lumpy fat deposits, over the thighs in particular, had a condition called cellulite was popularized a few years ago. But microscopic studies show that *"cellulite" is nothing more than body fat*. These individuals, mostly women, simply have more fat cells in that location, and the cells tend to accumulate fat. In view of what is now known, it is likely that these cells have abundant alpha$_2$ receptors that encouraged fat storage. That is not a disorder, but a condition a person was born with.

Those Crazy Weight Tables

Is it healthy or unhealthy to gain weight with age? That has been another long-running debate. Before the 1950s, it was customary to increase the desirable weight allowed with increasing age. But a lot of investigators began to ask questions about that, in part because it was quite clear that most people did not develop more muscles after age 25. The nonfat body did not increase in size. In point of fact, it often decreased as the years progressed. The increased weight that was being observed was mostly an increase in body fat. At the time, the United States and other industrialized nations were experiencing the post World War II epidemic of coronary heart disease. Early research implicated excess body fat as a factor in increasing a person's risk of having a heart attack or a stroke.

The Metropolitan Life Insurance Company used its data from the Build and Blood Pressure Study, Society of Actuaries, 1959, and constructed new height and weight tables for both men and women over age 25, without regard to increasing age. They did note the difference in desirable weights for different body frames. These new weight tables did not provide for gaining weight as you got older, but strengthened the concept that it was healthier to stay the same weight as the years went by, rather than to gain weight. The middle-aged spread was

Weight in Pounds
According to Frame (in Indoor Clothing).*

Desirable Weights for Men Aged 25 and Over			
Height with Shoes 1-inch Heels Feet Inches	Small Frame	Medium Frame	Large Frame
5 2	112-120	118-129	126-141
5 3	115-123	121-133	129-144
5 4	118-126	124-136	132-148
5 5	121-129	127-139	135-152
5 6	124-133	130-143	138-156
5 7	128-137	134-147	142-161
5 8	132-141	138-152	147-166
5 9	136-145	142-156	151-170
5 10	140-150	146-160	155-174
5 11	144-154	150-165	159-179
6 0	148-158	154-170	164-184
6 1	152-162	158-175	168-189
6 2	156-167	162-180	173-194
6 3	160-171	167-185	178-199
6 4	164-175	172-190	182-204

Desirable Weights for Women Aged 25 and Over			
Height with Shoes 2-inch Heels Feet Inches	Small Frame	Medium Frame	Large Frame
4 10	92-98	96-107	104-119
4 11	94-101	98-110	106-122
5 0	96-104	101-113	109-125
5 1	99-107	104-116	112-128
5 2	102-110	107-119	115-131
5 3	105-113	110-122	118-134
5 4	108-116	113-126	121-138
5 5	111-119	116-130	125-142
5 6	114-123	120-135	129-146
5 7	118-127	124-139	133-150
5 8	122-131	128-143	137-154
5 9	126-135	132-147	141-158
5 10	130-140	136-151	145-163
5 11	134-144	140-155	149-168
6 0	138-148	144-159	153-173

* For nude weight, deduct 5-7 lb (male) or 2-4 lb (female).
Prepared by Metropolitan Life Insurance Company. Derived primarily from data of the Build and Blood Pressure Study, Society of Actuaries, 1959.

no longer acceptable from a health point of view. These are still valuable tables, so I am including them here for those who want to use them.

After having used the Metropolitan Desirable Weight tables over 20 years, many heart specialists were astonished when, in 1983, the insurance company revised their tables. They actually allowed men to be 20 pounds heavier than before. This change was made because the Metropolitan Life Insurance Company observed from its latest statistics that individuals who were underweight did have a higher death rate. That was not inconsistent with observations made before the 1959 Metropolitan tables. In those earlier days, before the heart disease epidemic, the concern about being underweight was related to the frequency of tuberculosis and its resultant loss of weight. In 1900, tuberculosis was the leading cause of death in the United States, and myocardial infarctions were essentially unknown, In fact, the first heart attack in a living person was not described until 1908.

The reports about the increased death rates in people who were lean has caused a lot of confusion. This is apparent in the letter from a woman about her husband's attitude:

DEAR DR. LAMB: My husband is too fat! He is also stubborn and unwilling to do anything about it no matter what I tell him. His latest excuse for not getting on a diet and exercising is that thin people don't live as long as people who have a little "boar fat" around the middle. I think it is disgusting.

He claims that there are insurance reports that thin people have a shorter life expectancy. Is that true? I always thought that people who avoided being overweight lived the longest. Can you settle this argument? Maybe he will listen to you. I'm about ready to give up and plan how to spend his life insurance money.

The medical director for the Framingham Heart Study for the National Heart, Lung and Blood Institute, Dr. William Castelli, publicly recommended that doctors and nurses should not use the new 1983 Metropolitan tables. Using the Framingham data, he pointed out that in their experience the people who were underweight, and died, were cigarette smokers. Thus, the increased death rate in very thin people was associated with cigarette smoking, a known major risk factor for heart disease. Others supported Dr. Castelli's view.

Subsequent studies have shown that the low-weight subjects had a high death rate for the first few years of the study, then the death rate in the surviving light-weights was not increased or was actually less than the rest of the population. This supports the belief that many of the individuals with low body weights already had a significant disease, such as cancer, when they were first included in the study, and it was this unrecognized disease, not the low body weight, that increased the death rate in the next few years.

After this initial wave of criticism, the argument has died down, or at least been less public. In 1985 a panel of experts convened by the National Institutes of Health used the 1983 tables as a basis for recommendations on obesity. They concluded that if you weighed 20 pounds or more than provided by the 1983 tables that you should seek medical attention to help you control your weight. The 1983 Metropolitan Life Insurance Company weight tables are provided here for those who want to use this recommendation as a bench mark for the maximum they should weigh.

Since then the question of the best weight and which tables to use has been reviewed by investigators from the Harvard School of Public Health and affiliated institutions. They observed that most of the major studies used to establish ideal weights were flawed. A major flaw was failing to consider the influence of cigarette smoking. Another flaw was to eliminate from the evaluation the people who had diseases, such as heart attacks, that were related to being overweight. After reviewing all the studies and data they concluded that the 1959 Metropolitan weight tables do reflect the most ideal weight.

There has also been renewed interest in the importance in the distribution of excess body fat. Dr. Ulf Smith and colleagues of the University of Goteborg, Sweden, told an American Heart Association science writers' forum that abdominal obesity significantly increased the risk of heart attacks and strokes. He reinforced the adage that "the longer the waistline, the shorter the lifeline." From a health point of view, it is much worse to have abdominal obesity than fat around the hips. Since men are prone to abdominal obesity, and are more prone to heart attacks at earlier ages, that certainly fits with the concept. Dr. Smith found that women who were prone to male-type abdominal obesity were five times as likely to have high

Weight in Pounds
According to Frame (in Indoor Clothing).*

Desirable Weights for Men Aged 25 and Over

Height with Shoes 1-inch Heels Feet Inches		Small Frame	Medium Frame	Large Frame
5	2	128-134	131-141	138-150
5	3	130-136	133-143	140-153
5	4	132-138	135-145	142-156
5	5	134-140	137-148	144-160
5	6	136-142	139-151	146-164
5	7	138-145	142-154	149-168
5	8	140-148	145-157	152-172
5	9	142-151	148-160	155-176
5	10	144-154	151-163	158-180
5	11	146-157	154-166	161-184
6	0	149-160	157-170	164-188
6	1	152-164	160-174	168-192
6	2	155-168	164-178	172-197
6	3	158-172	167-182	176-202
6	4	162-176	171-187	181-207

Desirable Weights for Women Aged 25 and Over

Height with Shoes 2-inch Heels Feet Inches		Small Frame	Medium Frame	Large Frame
4	10	102-111	109-121	118-131
4	11	103-113	111-123	120-134
5	0	104-115	113-126	122-137
5	1	106-118	115-129	125-140
5	2	108-121	118-132	128-143
5	3	111-124	121-135	131-147
5	4	114-127	124-138	134-151
5	5	117-130	127-141	137-155
5	6	120-133	130-144	140-159
5	7	123-136	133-147	143-163
5	8	126-139	136-150	146-167
5	9	129-142	139-153	149-170
5	10	132-145	142-156	152-173
5	11	135-148	145-159	155-176
6	0	138-151	148-162	158-179

* From the 1983 Metropolitan Life Insurance Company desirable weight tables.

glucose levels, high blood pressure and diabetes than women with the typical hip and buttocks fat distribution.

None of these discussions really settle whether or not it is unhealthy to gain weight as you get older. But the National Institute on Aging now says that the ideal weights for both men and women do increase with age. As an example, a 5 foot 9 inch person's ideal weight when in the twenties is between 119 and 157 pounds (54 to 71 kilograms), but by age 60 to 69, the range is between 162 and 201 pounds (74 to 91 kilograms.)

Often the body mass index (BMI) is used to estimate whether a person is fat or lean. To find the BMI, the body weight in kilograms is divided by the height in meters squared. As an illustration, a person who is 5 feet 9 inches tall is 1.75 meters tall. If he weighs 160 pounds that is 72.72 kilograms. If you divide 72.72 by 1.75 squared (1.75 x 1.75 = 3.06) the BMI will be 23.76.

Can you use these tables or the body mass index to know what you should weigh? They are useful as a guide, but only a guide. They do not tell you how much of your body weight is fat and how much is nonfat. In almost all medical or health-related questions, *it is the amount of body fat that is important, not the actual weight.* There is a difference. A person who is very muscular and has very little body fat is different from another person who weighs the same, but has little muscle and a lot of fat. But no table is really applicable to everybody. This is apparent in this man's letter:

I read your discussion on body weight and health in *The Health Letter.* The weight tables seem not to help. I am 5 feet 9 and weigh 175 pounds. I have a medium frame, like most defensive backs who play football. I'm a competitive swimmer and recently took an electronic test which claimed I had 12 percent body fat. My chest is 43 and my waist 34. I'm 63. According to the tables my desirable weight is about 155. I have no idea how reliable the body fat test I took is. I suspect my body weight is normal, or rather what it should be, but I really don't know.

Ten years ago I was overweight—weighing 190 pounds. I started to swim seriously at that time. My weight has not significantly changed since I entered Master's Swimming competition seven years ago. I have taken weight exercises prescribed by my doctor which seemed to help my swimming. My basic question is, what should my weight be?

This man's weight is probably increased above the norm because of his exercise program. Not many people in the general population are involved in Masters Swimming competition or engage in regular strength training exercises that increase muscle weight.

Often, individuals who follow a strength training program and develop a lot of muscle with little fat will not fit on any of these tables. These people have to be considered in an entirely different manner. This man's letter is an example of what a person can do with such programs.

> DEAR DR. LAMB: What are the long term effects of weight lifting? I am a 31-year-old male and took up this hobby three years ago. At 205 pounds I would be considered by health insurance standards to be obese and have a shorter life span.
>
> Although I weigh 205, my waist is 34 inches, my chest is over 50 inches and thighs, 26 inches. I'm 5 feet 9 and have never felt better. My strength and endurance has tripled from what it was before I started this program. I take calcium and vitamin supplements and avoid fatty and fried foods, consume a lot of protein, egg whites but no yolks, lean meats, fish and fruits.
>
> Am I hurting my heart or bones? Does muscle weight have the same effect as fat weight?

The point I wish to make here is that this man will indeed appear overweight by most charts, tables and a body mass index, but unless it can be shown that an extra amount of the weight is fat, and if he has normal medical findings, his weight cannot be a problem. In fact he has increased his metabolically active tissue and that will help him avoid accumulating fat.

Another example of how important body composition rather than body weight can be is illustrated by one of the Apollo astronauts I examined.

I first evaluated this pilot when he was a candidate to become one of the Apollo astronauts. At age 20, he was 5 feet 11½ inches tall and weighted 154 pounds. I examined him when he was 30 years old and weighed 158 pounds. Only 17 percent of his body weight was fat, and you would have considered him to be lean and healthy. But his cholesterol level was 300, a significant evaluation. He began an exercise and diet program, and at age 32 his weight was 155 pounds, but only 9 percent of his body weight was fat. That meant he had gained muscle with his exercise program and lost body fat. His cholesterol had stabilized at 167, well below the levels that are associated with any increased risk of fatty-cholesterol deposits in his arteries. Notice that he would have checked out on height-weight tables, or the body mass index, about the same when his body weight was 17 percent fat as when it was 9 percent fat. But in his case, the percent of fat made a great deal of difference in his cholesterol level.

Measuring Fat

The inability to measure body composition, or to know how many pounds of body weight are fat and how many pounds are nonfat body weight, has led to many different ways of trying to measure this. One of the oldest and still popular methods is to *measure your skinfold*. It is a little more sophisticated than "pinching an inch." About half of the body fat is under the skin, and the rest is inside the abdomen and various tissues. This makes an estimate of the amount of fat under the skin a fairly reliable measurement of body fat. Several different sites have been recommended for skinfold measurements. The back of the arm is often used. A location on the abdomen, just above the pelvic brim, is a good location for abdominal fat.

There are also a number of newer methods designed to measure the fat thickness. These range from taking an X-ray to using ultrasound measurements.

A recent addition to methods of calculating body fat is to measure electrical impedance, the resistance to the flow of electrical current through the body. Electricity flows readily through salt water. Since your body is well over 50 percent salt water, it is a good conductor. Fat impedes the flow of electricity. The amount of fat is estimated by measuring electrical resistance to passing a small current through the body. The currently most widely used instruments attach electrodes to the wrists and ankles. A very small electrical current is passed through the body. Unfortunately, this method is not very reliable. There is too much variability. As the amount of water in the body fluctuates, so will the impedance. In general, the device tends to underestimate excess body fat and overestimate fat content in lean individuals.

Another method of measuring body fat is to immerse a person in water. The more body fat you have, the more you tend to float. The method really measures body density. It is not adaptable to regular office use or to follow a person's progress when losing weight.

Laboratories also measure the amount of body water by a variety of dilution techniques. One of these is the use of deuterated water, an isotope method which we used to determine how much body fat the astronaut I told you about had. That is how we knew that his body fat had decreased significantly. You could also tell it by physical examination of fat deposits under the skin.

One of the most accurate means of measuring percent of body fat is to measure the potassium content with a whole-body radiation counter. Unfortunately, this expensive device is found only in a few advanced research centers doing studies involving radiation.

How, then, can you tell how fat you are? You can pinch your skinfold and see how thick it is. You can strip and look at yourself in the mirror. You can try on some of your clothes you used to wear to see if you are gaining or losing. Your direct examination is about as good as you really need, along with remembering what you weighed when you were 25 years old. The "normal" range usually given for percent of body weight as fat is 15 to 20 percent for men and 20 to 25 percent for women. You can have a lot less body fat than that and be in optimal health. I studied the pentathletes who were in training to compete in the olympics and the average percentage of their body weight as fat was only 11 percent. Many were much lower than that. The lowest value was in one of the top athletes who had a percent body fat of only 6.4 percent. I might add that these young men were among the healthiest individuals I have examined.

Summary 6

1. You can get fat because of inherited characteristics, or you can get fat because of what you eat and not getting enough activity. Some people have both problems.
2. You are born with a life script that determines what you should weigh, and how fat you should be, at various stages of your life.
3. There is a strong tendency to inherit characteristics that control where you have body fat deposits.
4. Men tend to develop fat over the abdomen. Women tend to develop fat over the thighs and buttocks.
5. You have one type of fat cells that stores fat and resists releasing

fat. These special fat cells cause the persistent fat deposits, such as the "love handles" around the waist. Your other fat cells behave differently and you lose fat from them first when you are losing calories.

6. Spot reducing exercises do not work.
7. Cellulite is just body fat. Because of their location, these fat cells are commonly the kind that resist giving up their fat stores.
8. Unless low body weight is associated with a disease—which may not be recognized—or some degree of starvation, the nonsmoking person with the lowest body weight tends to live the longest.
9. Abdominal obesity is significantly associated with an increased risk of heart attacks and strokes.
10. Body weight tables are useful guides, but they do not separate body weight from body fat. It is the amount of body fat that is important.

Chapter 7

Some Medical Reasons to Lose Weight

So you have some extra pounds, do you need to lose them? Maybe not. If you want to lose weight for appearance, that is a personal choice. You should be aware that losing too much weight, or being too thin, is unhealthy.

Other than just for appearance, there are also some very good medical reasons to avoid being overweight. *But don't lose weight, just because you think you need to. Find out the status of your health before starting a weight losing program.*

One of the most important reasons to lose body fat is to avoid fatty-cholesterol deposits in the arteries that result in heart attacks, strokes and other medical problems. *Eliminating excess body fat is often one of the very best ways to lower the total cholesterol level.* Here again you need to individualize a weight control program. If a person already has an optimally low total cholesterol level and the various cholesterol fractions are in a good range, this is not an indication to go on a program to lose weight. Put another way, there is no reason to take penicillin for syphilis if you don't have syphilis, and there is no reason to go on a weight reduction program to lower your total cholesterol if it is already at an optimal level. But there is solid evidence that a high total cholesterol level will significantly increase a person's risk of a heart attack, and when it is high, a person needs to lose any excess body fat he or she has.

Abnormal cholesterol levels are not just a matter of body weight. Inherited characteristics influence the cholesterol levels as does diet, exercise, sex and any number of factors. Some invividuals are quite

81

lean and still have high total cholesterol levels. Most of these people inherited the characteristic. Other people are quite overweight and have low optimal levels of total cholesterol.

What are the cholesterol levels that should call for considering a diet to lose excess pounds of body fat? The first important value is the total cholesterol level. Current thinking is that the optimal level should be less than 200 mg per 100 ml of blood serum or plasma. Higher levels are equated to a moderate and high risk of having a heart attack. In general, the higher your total cholesterol level is above 200, the greater your risk of having a heart attack. An example of a man who should be on a diet that includes weight loss is described by his wife.

> DEAR DR. LAMB: Can you send me some information on a diet to prevent heart attacks and any ideas on how I can get my husband to realize that he can and will die of a heart attack if he continues his present lifestyle?
>
> He is 5 feet 9, weighs 185 pounds and is only 34. But his cholesterol is 325 and his father died of a heart attack at age 56. He loves red meat. He thinks because he doesn't eat snacks, cookies and cake that he is eating well. He has a real stressful job. At least he doesn't smoke!
>
> We have three small children and I am very worried about him.
>
> I try to cook healthy foods at home, but he travels half the time and apparently eats whatever he wants on the road. I have cut down on serving red meats, but he says he doesn't feel "full" without it. What can I do to help him change?

At 5 feet 9 and 185 pounds this man probably has room to lose a lot of body fat. A loss of 30 pounds of body fat could make a great deal of difference in his total cholesterol level. You never know this until a diet has been given an adequate trial. That means staying on the diet even when you are away from home. While a low-fat, low-saturated fat, low-cholesterol diet is important, such a diet is also a low-calorie diet. The associated weight loss in many cases is essential in correcting elevated total cholesterol levels.

An intake of excess calories of any origin is processed by the liver and converted to fat and cholesterol. These are combined into fatty-cholesterol particles which increases a person's risk of coronary heart disease.

Measuring your total cholesterol level is not enough. Other measurements are equally or more important in determining your risk and your need to lose excess pounds of body fat. Cholesterol really doesn't float around in your blood in a free form because it is a lipid, meaning fat-like, and it cannot be dissolved in water or blood. Nature has solved this problem by combining cholesterol, triglycerides and a blood protein. Triglycerides are simply fat, as discussed before. They are not soluble in water either. But blood proteins are, and by combining the protein with the fat and cholesterol a soluble fatty-cholesterol particle is formed. These fatty-cholesterol particles are called lipoproteins. Although you hear about cholesterol all the time, the real interest is in the lipoproteins that carry the cholesterol. When your total cholesterol is measured, it is really an index of the amount of fatty-cholesterol particles you have in your blood. The smallest fatty-cholesterol particles contain the least fat (triglyceride) and they are the most dense. That is why they are called high density lipoproteins (HDL). These little fatty-cholesterol particles are the scavengers in your blood. They mop up cholesterol and take it back to your liver to be reprocessed or eliminated. They protect your arteries from fatty-cholesterol deposits. When the amount of cholesterol in the HDLs is measured, that indicates how many of these little particles you have. The more you have the better, and that is why the higher your HDL-cholesterol is, the less likely you are to have coronary heart disease. It is not the cholesterol itself that is "good" but the friendly little fatty-cholesterol particles.

You also have larger fatty-cholesterol particles and they contain more triglyceride. These are called low density lipoproteins (LDL). These are the bad fatty-cholesterol particles that do deposit in the walls of your arteries and cause arterial blockage. The less of these you have the better. These are particularly likely to be produced in some overweight people. When your LDL-cholesterol is measured, that provides information on how many larger and dangerous fatty-cholesterol particles you have.

You can have a low total cholesterol level and still be at risk of a heart attack if your HDL-cholesterol level is low. It is generally stated that men should have at least 45 mg and women 55 mg of HDL-cholesterol per 100 ml of blood serum or plasma. Again, higher values are helpful. It follows that if your total cholesterol is less than 200 and your HDL-cholesterol is over 55, you have no reason to lose weight to improve your total cholesterol level or raise your HDL-cholesterol level. The HDL-cholesterol level can be raised by exercise, certain dietary changes and some medicines.

Equally important in terms of whether you need to lose weight or not is your blood pressure. Literally speaking, the higher your blood pressure the greater your risk of having a heart attack or a stroke. High blood pressure is an especially important risk factor in causing strokes. The Committee on Detection, Evaluation, and Treatment of High Blood Pressure has defined normal blood pressure for anyone over 18 as no more than 140/85—140 mm Hg for the systolic or upper reading and 85 mm Hg for the diastolic or lower reading. But don't be confused by these arbitrary figures. The truth is that the greater your pressure over 120/75 the greater your risk of heart attacks and strokes.

Just losing a few pounds of excess body fat seems to significantly lower blood pressure in many people, even when a person doesn't appear to be obese by usual standards. The loss of all or most of the excess pounds of body fat will often produce a dramatic improvement in blood pressure levels.

But accumulated body fat is not the only factor causing high blood pressure. Despite weight loss, the blood pressure may stay high. I was amused by the letter I received from a man who found this out with his personal experience.

DEAR DR. LAMB: I read your column about the value of becoming lean, trim and fit to control high blood pressure. You may be interested in my experience. About 14 years ago I read a famous book, *Aerobics*, and thought it meant that if a severe hypertensive who was overweight and not in good shape worked himself into good shape, he could eliminate his medicine.

The book said, "get yourself in superb physical condition and go see your doctor a year later and he will be amazed at your condition."

I started running and worked up to 3 1/2 miles. I lost many pounds and became quite slim and really felt in great shape. I discontinued taking my hypertensive medicines for many months. I ran easily with no strain and could have run much farther but decided at age 54 this was far enough.

After a year I went to see my doctor. He was amazed all right! My blood pressure was 240/140. He almost had a stroke when I told him I had run 3 1/2 miles that very morning.

He put me back on medication, but didn't tell me to stop running.

I'm still in good shape but now just do long walks almost every day and am also one of the world's oldest weight lifters—light weights, nothing over 140 pounds. I am still on medication. At age 69 I'm in remarkably good health except for my blood pressure.

This man's letter shows how much many people can do despite significant medical problems. It also shows that despite an outstanding exercise program and weight loss that the underlying medical problem may persist. It is a good example of why no one should stop his medicines prescribed by his doctor unless his doctor advises it.

Happily, many people who lose weight and improve their habits will lower their blood pressure, as this man's letter tells us.

DEAR DR. LAMB: I wanted you to know that your comments about alcohol and high blood pressure were right on target. While in the marines I was admitted to the Navy's Alcohol Rehabilitation Service. I was more than 30 pounds overweight and had been taking medicine prescribed for high blood pressure. I was told to lay off salt, and the alcohol was stopped, I was also put on a mild exercise program.

In the first three months my weight came down to 13 pounds below my allowed maximum. I was taken off blood pressure medication and my overall health soared.

I retired a year later and now go to school full time. I still don't drink and don't use table salt. I eat what I want, but try to use common sense, and my weight has stayed down and my blood pressure has improved even more.

I can't remember or imagine any benefit from alcohol which could equal the overall good feeling that I experience today.

There may be more than one factor affecting this man's health. The alcohol alone could have caused high blood pressure. But the fact that his blood pressure continued to improve long afterward suggests that the weight loss as well as salt restriction played an important role. Notice that, in his case, with the weight loss and other measures, he was able to stop his medicines and continued to have improvement in his blood pressure.

You can be overweight, eat the wrong foods and still have a low total cholesterol as this man's case shows.

DEAR DR. LAMB: My husband, age 53, is about 20 to 30 pounds overweight and his blood pressure fluctuates from normal to as high as 180/110. He controls it by bicycling 8 to 15 miles, two to three times a week, weather permitting. Otherwise he lives a sedentary, stress-filled life. Yet, his cholesterol count is only 165, so our doctor has told me that my husband can eat all the big bowls of ice cream he wants. Well, he's been eating ice cream before he goes to bed, every night, for the past 15 to 20 years, plus two large milk shakes a week. He consumes a half gallon of ice cream in five to six days. The rest of his diet is also very high in fats. Our doctor reported that my husband's blood circulation is excellent. However, he has deep creases in his ear lobes and often doesn't seem to be able to follow the simplest conversation. Is it possible for him to have hardening of the arteries to his brain despite a low cholesterol count? Are the creases in the ear lobes a good indicator of decreased blood flow to the brain?

While this man need not lose weight to lower his total cholesterol, it might be very helpful in terms of lowering his blood pressure. A crease in the ear lobe has not proved to be a good indicator of poor circulation, but high blood pressure is certainly a major risk factor for strokes because of damage to the arteries to the brain. It is more important in terms of stroke risk than a high total cholesterol. So, despite his low total cholesterol, this man has an indication for losing body weight. Since his exercise level is good, that means decreasing his calorie intake. The problem with the ice cream in his case is not its saturated fat content, but its high calorie content, which of course is from its fat and sugar content.

What if your cholesterol levels are in the optimal range and your blood pressure is also in a low optimal range? Then you don't need to go on a diet to improve either of these risk factors. You already have the optimal values that weight loss would produce.

One of the ways, then, to find out if you really need to lose body fat or not, is to have your total cholesterol, your HDL-cholesterol and your blood pressure measured. Then you can make a decision on the basis of facts that are significant to your health. There is some evidence that being obese, even without factors that increase your risk, will in itself increase your risk slightly.

While much is said about losing weight to lower total cholesterol and blood pressure to prevent heart disease, it is equally important for people who already have coronary heart disease and who are overweight. Such measures are important for people who have had a coronary bypass operation. Often the success of such operations really depends on what kind of preventive program a person follows after the operation. If a person has pain from heart disease, weight loss is often a major factor in treatment. The following letter describes a typical example of a person who needs to lose weight because of heart pain.

DR. LAMB: I have trouble walking even one block before I have to stop and rest, sometimes I hold on to a stop sign or whatever is near. After I've rested for just a few minutes I can keep walking again.

I get a tired, nauseous feeling and it usually affects my right arm, which gets tired and clammy. This happens sometimes when I make my bed or even when I hang clothes on the clothes line or when I walk a short distance. I have walked to town, about four blocks from my home, and have had to stop along the way. Does this sound like there is a problem? I had a heart problem 10 years ago and again 5 years ago. My doctor said it was a heart attack and left damage to the tip of my heart.

Can you tell me what I'm up against? My doctor called it angina and I'm hoping you can tell me what angina is. Should I be on medication? I know I'm overweight, but I find it difficult to lose even five pounds. I weigh 170 pounds and am 5 feet 1. I get this even when I walk very slow and I stay away from walking uphill.

Obviously this woman should be seeing her doctor. Losing weight would certainly help, not only to lower her cholesterol levels if they are elevated, or her blood pressure if it is high, but to decrease the work of the heart. She has angina pain because she doesn't have enough blood flow to allow her heart to increase its work very much. A significant decrease in body weight would help in terms of less angina and permit her to be more active. At that point, the increased activity could significantly improve her heart condition.

Some people who have extra pounds of body fat also have high blood glucose levels. Weight reduction often changes this. According to a Swedish study, a 50-year-old man, who has just a few extra pounds of body fat, may increase his risk of developing diabetes and high blood pressure in the following 10 years.

One of the interesting studies of the effect of diet and exercise was carried out by Dr. Kerin O'Dea of the Department of Medicine, University of Melbourne, Australia. He studied ten middle-aged Australian aborigines who had lived the Western lifestyle, including a diet of fatty meats, carbonated drinks and alcohol. All were obese, had high blood pressure and were diabetic. They returned to the hunter-gatherer lifestyle and ate only what they could hunt, fish or collect. Their diet included kangaroo, crocodile and turtle. They all lost weight steadily and at two months their blood glucose level had fallen and their glucose tolerance was improved. Their diet averaged only 1,200 calories a day and their physical activity was greatly increased. By seven weeks their blood clotting tendency was decreased as measured by bleeding times and the triglycerides (fat) level in the blood had fallen to normal.

Notice the combination of three problems, high blood pressure, obesity and diabetes. The increased bleeding time with weight loss is interesting, as one aspirin every other day to decrease a blood clotting tendency has been shown to significantly decrease the risk of heart attacks. It would appear that weight control in some individuals may have a similar benefit on blood clotting mechanisms.

Being overweight may also increase your risk of cancer. The American Cancer Society study, involving over a million people, shows that obese males are more prone to cancer of the colon, rectum and prostate gland. Obese women have a higher risk of cancer of the gall bladder, breast, uterus and ovaries.

In view of the relationship of being overweight to heart disease, strokes, cancer and diabetes, it is not surprising that individuals of normal body weight live longer than those who are overweight. The decrease in life span seems to be particularly true in men and women who are overweight before 50 years of age. This suggests that it is especially important to avoid being overweight at a young age.

Besides the dangers of high blood pressure, heart attacks, strokes and diabetes, there are other health risks from being overweight. Surgery is often more difficult and associated with more complications—some of which are life threatening—in people who are overweight compared to people of normal weight.

When you consider all these points, it becomes clear that there is no one rule about body weight that applies to everyone. If you are on the heavy side, it probably is wise to slim down, if you don't harm yourself by overdoing it. Before you begin any program, it is a good idea to really know your health status. If you already have optimal health findings, except for a few extra pounds of fat, you may not need to lose weight at all. In fact, it could be dangerous. It is an individual matter.

Summary 7

1. One medical reason to lose body fat is to lower an elevated total cholesterol and reduce your risk of a heart attack or other complications of fatty-cholesterol blockage of arteries.

2. People do inherit the tendency to have high total cholesterol levels and you can be of normal weight or even thin and have a high level.

3. An optimal total cholesterol level in terms of risk of having a heart attack is 200 mg or less.

4. An intake of excess calories of any origin: carbohydrate, protein, fat or all three, may cause your liver to form excess fatty-cholesterol particles.

5. Cholesterol is not soluble in water and cannot exist alone in your blood. It is combined with triglycerides (fat) and a blood protein to form lipoproteins which are soluble.

6. The small fatty-cholesterol particles (high density lipoproteins) are beneficial and protect against artery blockage. The HDL-cholesterol portion of your total cholesterol is a measure of how many of these protective particles you have.

7. The larger fatty-cholesterol particles (low density lipoproteins) cause artery blockage and the LDL-cholesterol portion of your total cholesterol is a measure of how many of these harmful particles you have.

8. Men should have at least 45 mg of HDL-cholesterol and women should have at least 55 mg of HDL-cholesterol.

9. If your total cholesterol level is less than 200 mg and your HDL-cholesterol is over 55 mg, there is no reason to diet to change these values.

10. If your blood pressure is elevated and you are overweight, you should lose any body fat you can. This often significantly lowers blood pressure.

11. An optimal blood pressure that is associated with the least risk of

a heart attack or stroke should be below 120/75, although most
doctors accept a value of 140/85 or less as normal.

12. You can have high blood pressure and not be overweight and it
can be on an inherited basis.

13. Decreasing body weight is often helpful to people who already
have heart disease and may help increase such a patient's exercise
capacity and freedom from pain.

14. Weight reduction may also improve diabetes or even correct it
entirely.

15. Being overweight also increases a person's risk of certain cancers.

16. Overweight people are prone to have more complications from
surgery than people of normal weight.

Chapter 8

Don't Be a Victim of Undernutrition

There are millions of people in the United States who are suffering from undernutrition because they have been on an unwise diet program. Most of their problems go unrecognized. There are many disorders and diseases that occur from malnutrition, including all the disorders associated with vitamin and mineral deficiencies, but the problem of simple calorie undernutrition in the adult is less evident and often develops insidiously. One of the unfortunate developments of the emphasis on being thin is undernutrition. You commonly hear that you should not be on a diet that contains less than 1,200 calories. That figure enables one to put together a balanced diet that should meet all the vitamin, mineral and protein requirements for the body's needs, *but it may not provide all the calories a person needs.* Some people restrict their calories below this level and still can't lose weight. Usually, these individuals are not supposed to be thin.

Normal Weight but Undernourished

Many people find that after losing weight—particularly if they have been on one of the quickie fad diets—they regain their weight just as soon as they eat a normal, healthy diet. They claim that they do not eat more than other people and that if they eat normally they gain weight. This lady expresses some of the frustration these people feel.

DEAR DR. LAMB: I am one of those women who gain weight by looking at food. I'm trying to convince my doctor that I am different from other women who do not have a weight problem, and I cannot

91

keep my weight off unless I stay on a low calorie diet. He doesn't believe me and thinks I eat more than I admit to. Do you have any information that would help me convince him that I'm telling the truth?

The idea that people were overweight because of eating too much has been a firmly held belief for a long time. I recall that when I was a medical student one of our professors emphatically told us that all fat people were liars when it came to their diet. He went on to say that almost all fat women had a candy bar in their purse. These attitudes simply reflect a lack of understanding of what causes a person to be overweight according to the charts and our ideas of what being overweight really is.

If you have to make heroic efforts to be thin, usually you are fighting your body. Faust, and his colleagues at Rockefeller University, studied obese people by putting them on a reducing regime, in the hospital, to the point where their body weight was normal. But despite normal body weight their metabolism was not normal. They needed 25 percent fewer calories than comparable individuals of the same weight who had never been obese to avoid regaining their weight. It really is true that some overweight people don't need many calories. *For those people to lose fat, they have to be on a very-low-calorie diet, that can have an adverse effect on their health.*

Scientists from Kings College University of London also studied the differences in energy requirements between 16 women who had been obese and lost weight and 16 women who matched them in age and weight but had never been overweight (*American Journal of Clinical Nutrition*, 45: 1987, 914). The formerly obese women used an average of only 1,289 calories a day but their lean counterparts used an average of 1,945 calories a day. Whether the women were exercising, resting or sleeping, the formerly obese women used fewer calories than their never-obese counterparts. This points up the fact that despite losing body fat, the basic reason for the original weight gain persisted. If the formerly-obese women started eating as much as their never-obese counterparts, they would regain their weight. The only way the two groups of women could continue to weigh the same and to eat the same would be if something happened to increase the calorie requirements of the formerly-obese women.

As a person who is supposed to carry more fat gains the weight he or she is programed to carry, the daily calorie requirements increase. That is because it takes more energy to move a heavier body and more energy is required to run a larger body. A point of balance is reached, where the weight of the person is such that the calorie requirements match the calories consumed, and the weight stabilizes at that level.

Hirsch and colleagues studied a group of women and one man who were members of Overeaters Anonymous. All had weighed more than 200 pounds and then reduced to normal weights. When the researchers studied their fat cells, they observed that they were tiny. The women did not menstruate. They had low levels of thyroid hormone. Remember, if you starve yourself, the body decreases the amount of active thyroid hormone it produces so you can survive a period of starvation. These individuals exhibited the characteristics often seen in young, thin girls suffering from anorexia nervosa, the problem of self-starvation. In short, even though these people were of normal weight and external appearance, they were suffering from undernutrition.

This problem is particularly apt to occur in middle-aged women. Just as puberty causes changes in body fat deposits in women, the middle-aged phase of life often causes another change. Many women find this undesirable because it does alter their appearance. At that point some go to heroic lengths to try to retain the body-shape they had when they were in their early twenties. They want to fit the body-image they have of themselves. The result is semi-starvation or undernutrition.

Just as a person may gain weight and eventually achieve a balance between calories required and calories consumed, the same thing can happen with undernutrition. As a person loses weight, the calorie requirements diminish while the energy system is being shut down. Eventually the starved body uses no more calories than the small amount consumed and a new level of calorie balance is achieved — but at the expense of losing the higher level of energy capacity and often at the expense of a person's health.

To use an example of how this works, consider the hypothetical situation of a person who weighs 200 pounds and consumes 3,000 calories a day to maintain his body weight. That person is in energy balance at that weight and that calorie intake. If this person then reduces his calorie intake to 1,500 calories a day, he will have a negative calorie balance and will start losing weight. As his weight falls, his calorie requirements also decrease. Eventually, say at 140 pounds, his body will require only the 1,500 calories a day to be in the same energy equilibrium. At that point his body weight will stabilize and he will not lose any more weight despite consuming half as many calories as he once did when he weighed 200 pounds. This is one reason why many people on calorie restricted diets find that the longer they stay on the diet, the less effective it is in terms of weight loss, and eventually it no longer induces weight loss at all.

Now if this same individual returns to consuming 3,000 calories a day, he will be in positive calorie balance and will start gaining weight. As he gains weight, his calorie requirements will increase. Eventually his calorie requirements will equal his intake of 3,000 calories a day and he will stop gaining weight.

The Minnesota Experience

One of the studies that has left a lasting impression on me was one done at the University of Minnesota by Dr. Ancel Keys and his colleagues in the late 1940s. The study showed how damaging even a 1,570 calorie a day diet can be. The diet contained 50 grams of protein, 30 to 45 grams of fat and 300 grams of carbohydrate. It included vitamins, and was in all respects a balanced diet.

The study involved 32 young healthy men of an average age of 25.5 years. Previously, they had been in calorie balance by consuming 3,490 calories a day. They were not fat and they were very active. These young men were studied for 12 weeks while on a 3,490 calorie diet, followed by 24 weeks on the 1,570 calorie diet, and then again for 12 weeks on the original diet. Each subject had a job that required 15 hours of work a week and was required to walk outside 22 miles a week. In addition, each subject walked for 30 minutes on a treadmill each week. At the end of 24 weeks on the reduced-calorie diet, they had lost about 25 percent of their body weight.

Of course, losing 25 percent of their body weight was evident physically. They had a wasted facial appearance and were emaciated. There were other widespread changes. Their skin was cold. After all, their body was doing everything it could to prevent loss of calories through the skin. The skin was even slightly bluish. That indicates a marked decrease in blood flow through the skin, which caused the blood to give up more oxygen than usual. The decreased circulation was a normal adaptation to limit heat loss through radiation and convection. There was evidence of a decrease in growth, as indicated by a slower than usual growth of hair and fingernails. Some had a significant loss of hair, which can occur if you restrict your calories too much. They did not have the calories needed to support anabolic metabolism to form new tissue. When they had a cut or wound, it healed slowly. Healing requires protein formation or an anabolic process.

Not surprisingly, these subjects felt cold all the time, even when the temperature was warm. That, too, is part of the picture of decreased blood flow through the skin. The sensation of feeling cold is a symptom you can watch out for when you are on a reducing diet. It indicates that your skin is conserving heat because you do not have any calories to spare.

As metabolism slows, there is less demand for oxygen. That decreases the amount of blood the heart has to pump. That is useful in some medical situations when you need to decrease the work load on the heart, but it is not healthy in normal circumstances. The heart rate in these young men slowed because of this. Of course, they were very active physically, which will slow the heart rate, also.

As occurs because of a diet grossly deficient in calories, they lost salt and water. The combination caused them to have symptoms of faintness and giddiness. Here again is a symptom that occurs often on fad diets, particularly those that eliminate carbohydrates. The salt and water loss also led to a susceptibility to muscle cramps. However, muscle cramps, too, may be related to the decrease in cold tolerance. Individuals who have lost weight to the point of having a low cold tolerance may well have lower leg temperatures at night, which contributes to developing leg cramps.

These young men had digestive complaints, including gas, colic and diarrhea. There were changes in the functions of their endocrine glands, and a loss in sex drive. When you are lean because of suffering from undernutrition, you are not more sexy but less sexy. They also had personality changes, characterized by a sharp decrease in spontaneous activity and a tendency to withdraw. Their work capacity, as measured during the treadmill exercise, declined significantly.

The diet caused them to have fatigue. That is an important point, and the single most commonly experienced symptom by individuals on a diet overly restricted in calories. *Fatigue is the universal symptom of undernutrition*, unless you are taking appetite suppressants that are really pep pills or "uppers" which mask the effect.

These young men were not through with their difficulties the day the restricted diet ended. It took them six months to recover from the experience. They continued to feel tired and have a low sex drive for months afterward, even though they were consuming a super-high-calorie diet.

These young men were different from overweight individuals simply because they did not have an excess body fat problem to begin with. And most people do not do the level of physical work these young men continued to perform, despite dietary restrictions. Nevertheless, there are plenty of individuals on very low-calorie diets who are out on the jogging trail or on the handball court, expending as much or more effort than these young men did. I have received many letters from wives complaining about their husbands having lost interest in them since becoming engrossed in an exercise program. The complaint is that they are not interested in sex any more, and the reason is not just because they are running, but because they are running on an empty tank.

Even the person with extra pounds of body fat may have problems similar to those experienced by these young men, if the fat is necessary and intended to be there. Individuals who are designed to weigh 175 pounds, and insist on weighing 135, may look great in terms of measurements, but their machinery is in trouble, and they have usually lost their normal level of energy. There is not as much zip in the motor because they are running uphill on empty. The loss of energy and sense of well-being, along with other changes, are simply ignored in the quest to look young and thin.

There is an important point that needs to be made. Normally, 50 to 55 grams of good quality protein should be enough for an adequate diet. But when you limit your calorie intake below the number needed to sustain your normal body weight, you may need more protein. Why? Because your body will use the protein in your diet for calories, rather than to do such things as grow hair and fingernails. In order to avoid a protein deficiency, you must have both an adequate intake of calories and an adequate intake of good quality protein. Why not just increase the protein and keep the calories low? It won't work as long as your body needs calories. There is nothing sacred about protein. It provides calories for energy the same as do carbohydrates and fats.

When you see what happened to these young, healthy men on a 1,570 calorie diet, you realize that those 1,200 calories a day diets can cause real problems. There are millions of Americans who go on diets that provide no more than 1,200 calories. Many actually are on diets that provide even fewer calories. I receive letters from some people who have decreased their calorie intake to 600 to 800 calories a day.

Whenever you go on a severe, calorie-restricted diet, your body starts shutting the metabolic system down. One of its compensatory mechanisms is to decrease the amount of active metabolic tissue. That means losing muscles and other nonfat tissues. In simple terms, if you are smaller, you need less energy. This happened to the young men in Minnesota and they achieved a new, lower calorie balance, but they were not healthy.

Lessons from Anorexia Nervose

Anorexia nervosa is an extreme example of undernutrition caused by psychopathology. It occurs when a person, usually a young girl, develops an obsession with being thin. She usually has a false body image. Even when she is thin, she looks in the mirror and thinks of herself as being fat. The loss of weight is usually the first sign the parents see. It may be rapid, with a decrease in weight from 120 pounds to 75 pounds in a matter of months. She is often emaciated, apathetic, weak and depressed. She may be in danger of committing suicide. Her personality changes, she becomes withdrawn and resists efforts to help her. A typical case is described by this mother.

DEAR DR. LAMB: I have an 18-year-old daughter who still lives at home. She has always been a normal weight teenager, but in the past four months she has lost a lot of weight. I feel she is much too thin. She is 5 feet 5 inches tall and weighs about 92 pounds.

I asked her about her weight and she tells me she is fat and needs to lose weight. I can't even get her to eat more than a few bites. She keeps telling me I'm overreacting and I should leave her alone. Should I? If I do will she stop? Is she sick? I'm very concerned.

The girl's statement that she needs to lose weight, despite her low weight for her height, is typical of a false body image. Leaving the girl alone will not help, as she needs to resolve her basic psychological problems, since she is doing real damage to herself.

Not all of these changes seen in patients with anorexia nervosa are because of undernutrition. Some of them are related to the fundamental psychopathology. In addition to the severe weight loss, anorexia nervosa victims will have other changes that are the result of undernutrition. Fatigue, and loss of energy to engage in spontaneous activity, are prominent. The skin feels cold. There is that sign again of closing down the skin's air conditioning effect to conserve energy. The metabolic system is shut down to the point where there is little need to eliminate calories of heat. Like the young men from Minnesota, the patient may have skin that is bluish in color, despite being in a warm room. There is evidence of loss of fat deposits, including wasting of the breasts, buttocks and other areas of normal fat deposits in the female. In addition, she will have a loss of interest in sex and will stop menstruating because of associated hormonal changes. Similar changes are also seen in the male with anorexia nervosa. He, too, will have a loss in sexual interest and will experience changes in hormonal levels associated with the function of the pituitary-gonad endocrine glands.

Undernutrition in young people may have permanent effects. The skeleton is not fully mature until after 30 years of age, despite the fact that growth in height has stopped. Remember, you must have enough calories to permit the proteins in your diet to be used for growth. Bone development requires calcium, but it also requires protein. In the years when the skeleton is still developing, if there is not sufficient calories and protein, the bones will be somewhat like the fingernails and hair seen in the young men in the Minnesota experiment. There will be a failure in complete development. That leads to a smaller, weaker skeleton than the individual should have, making it more likely to develop osteoporosis and skeletal deformities later in life. In severe cases, young women will already have loss of bone and even bone fractures from osteoporosis occurring long before the time for the menopause. Calcium deficiencies, protein deficiencies, calorie deficiencies and resulting loss of function of the sex glands with decreased production of estrogen cause this condition in these young girls. *Good nutrition in early life is essential to prevent unwanted changes in middle and later life.*

Undernourished Athletes

It is important to realize that undernutrition can be serious. *Even in people you think are healthy, undernutrition can be fatal.* This has been seen in a number of lean marathon runners who have had unexplained deaths. Because of the energy used in marathon running, and the limits on calorie intake to maintain a low body weight—theoretically to improve their performance—they suffered from undernutrition. Severe states of undernutrition can upset the chemical balance of the body and may cause a loss of potassium from the cells. When such mineral changes occur, they can cause irregularities of the heart. Some of these may be fatal. The moral is, even if you are an endurance athlete, like a marathoner, it is not wise to push your body into a severe calorie deficit.

Undernutrition in young women can lead to loss of normal menstrual functions. This need not be just from limiting calories, but may be associated with a high level of physical activity as well. It is important to realize that undernutrition really means not consuming enough calories to meet your body's healthy demands. When you increase your demands, your body needs more calories. If your level of calorie requirements are high enough, you can starve yourself, despite having what you might consider an adequate calorie intake—as happened to the young men in the Minnesota experiment. It is the calorie balance that counts, not the absolute number. A state of undernutrition can occur, even if the negative calorie balance is small, if it persists over a period of time. The fact that it is a gradual loss does not mean it is safe or healthy. No matter how you get there, a state of undernutrition is an unhealthy state.

Undernourished Societies

Chronic undernutrition is frequently seen in societies where there is a persistent food shortage. These people are often said to suffer from protein-calorie malnutrition. This can have many adverse effects on the children, but it also affects the adults. In regions where the adult male must engage in agricultural practices to survive, he must work hard but has very little to eat. He is forced into some of the same circumstances that people in more affluent societies impose upon themselves. In many ways he is like the young men in the Minnesota experiment.

These adult males can only expend a limited amount of energy because of their undernutrition, and therefore have a suboptimal work performance. That limits their opportunity to be productive. In turn, that perpetuates their undernutrition. It becomes a vicious cycle that has many sociological implications. The low energy level of people in this situation has a lot to do with their inability to interrelate with their family members and in community programs.

The women in such societies also suffer from undernutrition. They may not gain weight during a pregnancy, and that results in infants with low birth weights. The children have less than optimal development.

Undernutrition in the adult usually results in the individual being quite lean, even emaciated, but the most troublesome symptom is the loss of energy. *The first sign of undernutrition is this characteristic loss of energy and the inability to sustain prolonged physical work.* It is difficult to imagine how many adults in our privileged society actually are tired, their energy is at low ebb, simply because they are not consuming enough calories of energy to meet their body's daily requirements.

Decreased Work Capacity

There is a direct relationship between calories consumed and the physical work a person can do. This was evident in studies of the output of young German miners in World War II. When they consumed 2,800 calories a day, they cut 7.0 tons of coal, but when they consumed an additional 800 calories a day, they were able to cut 10 tons a day without losing body weight. This is a gross demonstration of the effects of calorie intake on performance capacity, which can be measured objectively, whereas the general sense of loss of energy is more subjective. Nevertheless, if you are on a weight-losing diet and find that you have lost your zest, perhaps you are a victim of undernutrition, and that is not good for your body or your mind.

Summary 8

1. Millions of people in affluent societies are suffering from under-

nutrition because they overly restrict their calorie intake.

2. Many "overweight" individuals are normally supposed to be that way. Excessive calorie limitation in these individuals causes a form of anorexia nervosa even though they may appear to be of normal weight after semi-starvation.

3. When a normally "overweight" individual loses his normal "extra" fat, that individual will require 15 to 25 percent fewer calories than might be expected in similar individuals who have never been overweight. It's true that they regain the weight they lost if they eat the same amount that similar "never-overweight" people consume.

4. As you gain weight, your energy requirements increase until they equal your calorie consumption. At that point your weight is stable for the level of calorie consumption.

5. As you decrease calorie intake you lose weight. As your weight decreases, your calorie requirements decrease. Eventually your calorie requirements match your calorie intake and you stop losing weight at that level of calorie consumption.

6. The longer you stay on a calorie restricted diet, the less effective it is in causing you to lose weight.

7. Healthy people who lose too much weight experience many health problems, including fatigue, personality changes, digestive complaints and a lack of sex drive and sexual ability.

8. If your diet does not provide enough calories, your body will use the protein in your diet for energy and you will effectively be on a protein deficient diet.

9. Individuals with anorexia nervosa suffer severe undernutrition which can be fatal.

10. Undernutrition up to age 30 can limit bone development and increase the risk of osteoporosis (dissolving bones) later in life. In extreme cases, severe undernutrition causes osteoporosis with fractures in young girls.

11. High levels of physical activity along with limited calorie intake can cause undernutrition even in athletes.

12. In some societies, the lack of available food results in undernutrition. This decreases the population's work capacity and affects the whole social structure.

13. Your calorie consumption directly affects your capacity for physical work.

Chapter 9

How Much of What Do You Need?

If young healthy people can suffer from undernutrition on a 1,570 calorie a day diet, how many calories do you need? It is important to realize that those calorie recommendations on most weight-losing diets are so arbitrary that they really cannot be an answer to your individual needs. That is the first thing that is wrong with most of the weight-losing diets promoted to the public. You need a proper evaluation to know how many calories you require, not an arbitrary figure. Your calorie needs are dependent upon many factors, not just a desire to lose weight. To maintain good health, your body needs as many calories as it uses every day. And how can you find our how many calories that is? By having your calorie needs measured.

Your Minimal Calorie Requirements

Unless you lived in a closed chamber that could either measure your heat production, or your oxygen consumption, you could not really measure your daily needs directly. The alternative is to make measurements that are related to it. One of the best of these is to measure your oxygen consumption for a short time interval, preferably early in the morning under resting conditions, while in the fasting state. You will really be measuring only your calorie needs for those conditions. Your requirements will increase as the day progresses and your body is more active. Nevertheless, this is a good bench mark to use in making an educated guess as to your real calorie requirements, rather than just using an arbitrary value provided by some diet. Remember your basics, and the point that for each liter of oxygen your body uses, you will have burned enough foodstuffs to equal approximately 4.825 calories.

If your oxygen requirements are measured for a specific time interval, that measure can be used to calculate how much oxygen you need for 24 hours under the same conditions, which I will call a near-basal state. It is a simple matter, then, to multiply the calories this represents for an hour by 24 for a 24-hour value. A person who uses 250 ml of oxygen a minute will use 360 liters in 24 hours. Multiply 360 by 4.825 and you will find that the near-basal requirements for 24 hours would be 1,737 calories. Clearly, this person cannot be on a 1,200 calorie diet and meet his daily calorie requirements. He will require more than 1,737 calories too, because he is not going to be in the near-basal state during all 24 hours. The only time he will need fewer calories per hour will be while he is sleeping. If a person only needed 225 ml of oxygen a minute, he would have a near-basal requirement of 1,563 calories. If he used 200 ml of oxygen a minute, he would need 1,389 calories. These are realistic figures for near-basal calorie requirements, and they explain why many low-calorie diets eventually result in undernutrition.

How can you get your near-basal oxygen requirements measured? That is the hardest part. Neither doctors nor weight control facilities are doing this. Doctors stopped doing it when they found better ways to measure thyroid function than the old classical basal metabolic rate (BMR) test. When I have referred to using the 4.825 factor in relation to oxygen utilization in my newspaper column, I have received many letters asking where you could get it done. Hopefully, it will be easier to get such a measurement when more people realize why it is so important to know more accurately, on an individual basis, how many calories a person requires.

At present, your best bet is to get your doctor to refer you to a doctor or laboratory that measures pulmonary functions. Most of these, because they measure your lungs' capacity to exchange air and provide oxygen, do have the equipment that can be used to measure oxygen consumption. Many cardiac laboratories that do cardiac catheterizations also have the equipment to do this. In fact, oxygen utilization is used to calculate how much blood the heart is pumping to deliver oxygen. Some exercise physiology laboratories will also be able to make such a measurement. At present, you can't just walk into your

doctor's office, or weight control center, and find out how many calories you need on the basis of your oxygen utilization. This measurement is very important to the person who needs to lose body fat, and
can't despite being on a restricted diet.

Another way to measure your near-basal calorie requirement is to
calculate it from your fat-free body weight. Remember that *fat under
the skin, around organs or around cells, is not part of your active
metabolic machinery that converts energy, or releases calories of heat.
While fat cells are not inactive, they do not contribute significantly to
the calorie exchange results.* The studies at the University of Minnesota established that in both males and females, between the ages of 20
and 60 years, *a kilogram of fat-free body weight used 4.4 ml of oxygen
a minute.* That is equivalent to 30.72 calories per 24 hours.

You can see how this works out by using the example of a 70-kilo-
gram (154-pound) person. If 20 percent of his body weight is fat, that
means his fat-free body weight is 56 kilograms. It follows that 56
times 30.72 calories per kilogram is 1,720 calories, and that would be
the near-basal calorie requirements for such an individual for 24
hours. If you want to manipulate figures, you will find this fits well
with the calculations based on measuring oxygen consumption in near-
basal conditions.

Earlier I showed you that Astronaut Ed White used 4,737 ml of
oxygen a minute when we tested him at maximum exertion, and that
meant he was momentarily using 1,371 calories an hour. At the time
we evaluated him for the astronaut program, he weighed 171 pounds
and was 13 percent body fat. That meant his lean body mass was 67.6
kilograms. At 30.72 calories per kilogram an hour, his near-basal energy requirements should have been 2,077 calories a day or 86.56
calories an hour. That is a high figure but he was a big lean man. That
means he was able to use nearly 16 times as many calories during
maximum effort as he normally used at near-basal levels.

Before you can use your fat-free body weight to calculate your calorie needs, you have to know what it is. To find that out, you have to
rely on the various methods to measure your percent of body fat, and
many of the methods commonly available are not that accurate. A
properly-done skinfold measurement, at enough proper sites on the
body, can provide a reasonable and practical approach to this problem.
There is a flip side to these relationships. You can use your near-basal
oxygen measurement to calculate your fat-free body weight. When

you know that, you can determine what percent of your body weight is fat and what percent is fat-free body weight.

Your Brain Has a Sweet Tooth

When you are at rest, your brain uses more calories than any other part of your body. It uses about 500 calories each 24 hours. Think about that. It uses almost a third of the energy used by your entire body under basal resting conditions. You may recall that the brain requires very little energy for even the most difficult mental task. That is true, but the brain needs lots of energy just to do all the other things it must do to operate your body. Remember that it monitors your body temperature and controls the blood flow through your skin and other parts of the body. It has to handle all the signals from the entire body and respond to them. All that automatic activity we never even think about, takes lots of energy. It's like needing a lot of electrical energy to run a powerful computer.

The brain is particular about what kind of energy it uses, too. It uses only glucose. During a 24-hour period, your brain will use 125 grams of glucose, or 500 calories. It uses only minute amounts of amino acids from protein to form trace amounts of brain chemicals, such as serotonin, but no fatty acids. Why? Because of the blood-brain barrier that limits what can get into the brain. Through a complex chemical mechanism, glucose can get through that barrier. Remember the theory about letting tryptophan into the brain to increase the serotonin level? The reason it is so tricky to get tryptophan into the brain is because that blood-brain barrier will not allow hardly any food item through, except glucose. It will allow alcohol to pass but the brain cells cannot use alcohol for energy. For the brain, alcohol is just a drug. Only the liver can metabolize alcohol.

What about people who are not eating any carbohydrates? That is another problem which I'll discuss in more detail later, but for now you need to know that when an abnormal product, called ketones, is formed in that situation, the brain can use them in place of glucose. Ordinarily, if you are healthy and on a satisfactory diet, you should not produce ketones.

The brain's requirements for glucose should tell you why your body needs carbohydrates under normal conditions. People often ask about "brain foods." The only real brain food is glucose.

Calories for Activities

Since you need calories to support your activities during the day, you will need more than your near-basal calorie requirements. If you could walk around all day, with a means of measuring your oxygen utilization, you would have the basis for a rather accurate assessment of your daily calorie requirements, including the calories required for your various activities. But that is not practical. As a substitute, the energy requirements for various activities have been estimated, and recommendations for daily calorie requirements are based on these. Usually, these measurements have been expressed as the calories used during the activity, so they include both your near-basal energy requirements and the energy required for your activities. That means they are extremely rough estimates that can be wide of the mark, but they do serve as a guide to know what you can expect your daily energy requirements to be. In any case, your daily calorie requirements should never be below your near-basal energy requirements for 24 hours, and that can be measured.

Most estimates assume that you will sleep eight hours a day, and that will use about 500 calories. More specifically, a 70-kilogram man will use about 540 calories during eight hours of sleep. Using the same man as a model, he will be engaged in about 12 hours of light activity, such as being seated or standing, and use 1,300 calories for that, or about 110 calories an hour. On average, he may engage in an hour of moderately heavy work, such as walking, cycling, dancing or other activities, which will require 300 calories used in 24 hours. That totals an average of 2,740 calories used in 24 hours. For a woman who weighs 58 kilograms (128 pounds), using similar calculations she will need 2,030 calories for 24 hours. Such calculations are the basis for some common recommendations that men weighing 70 kilograms will require 2,700 calories a day and women weighing 58 kilograms will require 2,100 calories a day.

Based on such calculations, the National Academy of Sciences' Food and Nutrition Board has made recommendations on calorie requirements for men and women of different ages, heights and weights. These, too, can only be used as a guide, because there is so much variation in what each person does. But they are instructive when you start thinking about going on a 1,200 calorie diet to lose weight and want to avoid undernutrition.

Mean Heights and Weights and Recommended Energy

	Age (years)	Weight (kg)	Weight (lb)	Height (cm)	Height (in.)	Energy Needs (calories)	Energy Needs (with range)
Males	15-18	66	145	176	69	2800	(2100-3900)
	19-22	70	154	177	70	2900	(2500-3300)
	23-50	70	154	178	70	2700	(2300-3100)
	51-75	70	154	178	70	2400	(2000-2800)
	76+	70	154	178	70	2050	(1650-2450)
Females	15-18	55	120	163	64	2100	(1200-3000)
	19-22	55	120	163	64	2100	(1700-2500)
	23-50	55	120	163	64	2000	(1600-2400)
	51-75	55	120	163	64	1800	(1400-2200)
	76+	55	120	163	64	1600	(1200-2000)
Pregnancy						+300	
Lactation						+500	

This is quite a maze of information to grapple with when you want to know how many calories you need a day. Nevertheless, it underscores how restrictive many diets are compared to a person's actual needs. In considering these many factors that affect your calorie balance, my own opinion is that your daily calorie intake should not be less than your near-basal energy requirements. If it were even that low, and you do anything besides lie in bed all day,, you are going to be in a negative calorie balance. Unless you are overweight because of consuming too many calories, that will gradually force you into a state of undernutrition. You only want to restrict your calories enough to enable you to eliminate pounds of body fat that you acquired because of bad eating habits and lack of activity. You want to stay within the range of your basic inherited script. That may not call for you to be super thin, the adult form of near anorexia nervosa.

Muscle Loss Can Make You Fat

You need to keep in mind that your near-basal calorie requirements may not tell the whole story, either. If you are already too thin and have been abusing your body with excessive calorie restriction and physical activity, your body will have shut down your metabolism to save you from yourself. That low metabolic level may result in measured near-basal calorie requirements that are actually below your optimal calorie intake.

As your body suffers from undernutrition and shrinks its fat-free weight, you lose active metabolic tissue. Remember the room with the furnace and the air conditioner analogy. Undernutrition decreases the size of the furnace by decreasing the amount of metabolically active, heat producing cells. That decreases your calorie requirement. Your body literally shrinks your metabolically-active tissues so you can survive despite consuming too few calories. That isn't healthy, and it will take a long time to regain your metabolically-active tissue by the anabolic process.

After your metabolically-active tissue has been shrunk, you will then require fewer calories to maintain your body weight. Your near-basal energy requirements will have been abnormally decreased. As a result, you will need to continue an inadequate diet to avoid gaining body fat. If your fat-free body is smaller, and therefore needs fewer calories, that leaves more calories to be stored as body fat. The awful truth is that unwise dieting can make it harder for you to avoid obesity in the future. On the contrary, as your fat-free body weight increases, from developing metabolically-active tissue, your daily calorie requirements increase and you can eat a better diet without gaining body fat. The main way you increase your metabolically-active tissue is to increase the size of your muscles. That is one reason why properly designed exercise programs are far superior to excessively restricted diets to help you obtain the proper weight.

Feed a Fever

Your calorie requirements can be greatly affected by your health. It is true that you should "feed a fever." As the body heats up with increased metabolism to raise your body temperature, you need to provide enough calories to meet the increased demands. When this doesn't happen, a person can develop a calorie deficit rather quickly. This can occur at any age. A sick child may need increased calories, but actually have his calories decreased because of fear of making his illness worse. The reason many people get emaciated with a chronic illness is not just because they don't eat much. Often, it is because the body's metabolism has been stepped up. A good example here is advanced tuberculosis. Despite a large calorie intake, patients with tuberculosis lose weight because their metabolism is increased, and they are releasing a lot of calories of heat through the skin. Considering the increased calorie demands of many illnesses, it is not surprising that hospitalized patients often lose a lot of weight. There is an increase in calorie demands after surgery, during the anabolic phase of healing. As any parent knows, growth requires an increased intake of calories. That is why teen-agers are constantly in the refrigerator or snacking.

Get Enough Protein

You need to consider more than total calories when you are planning your diet. You need to be sure you get enough good quality protein. As mentioned previously, you need to consume enough calories so your body doesn't need to use your protein for energy, but can use that protein in the many building requirements for the body. *Anyone on a diet that is inadequate in calories, and who does not have body fat stores available for energy, is on a protein-deficient diet.* That is why so many people on a calorie-deficient diet are said to suffer from a protein-calorie deficiency.

In 1977 the U.S. Senate Select Committee on Nutrition and Human Needs recommended that 15 percent of the total calories in the diet should come from protein, no more than 30 percent from fat, and the rest, 55 percent, from carbohydrates. That means if you were consuming 2,000 calories a day, 300 calories should be from protein. Since there are four calories per gram for protein you would need 75 grams of protein. If you were on a 1,500 calorie diet, 225 calories should be

---

**Food and Nutrition Board,
National Academy of Sciences –
National Research Council
Recommended Daily Dietary Allowances,**[a]
Revised 1980

*Designed for the maintenance of good nutrition of
practically all healthy people in the U.S.A.*

	Age (years)	Weight (kg)	Weight (lb)	Height (cm)	Height (in)	Protein (g)
Males	15-18	66	145	176	69	56
	19-22	70	154	177	70	56
	23-50	70	154	178	70	56
	51+	70	154	178	70	56
Females	15-18	55	120	163	64	46
	19-22	55	120	163	64	44
	23-50	55	120	163	64	44
	51+	55	120	163	64	44
Pregnant						+30
Lactating						+20

[a] *The allowances are intended to provide for individual
variations among most normal persons as they live in the
United States under usual environmental stresses. Diets
should be based on a variety of common foods in order to
provide other nutrients for which human requirements have
been less well defined.*

---

from protein, or 56 grams of protein. A 1,200 calories diet would provide only 180 calories or 45 grams of protein.

The Food and Nutrition Board, National Academy of Sciences-National Research Council's 1980 recommendations concerning protein intake were expressed as grams of protein needed for different age groups. Their recommendations are shown in the accompanying table.

Your diet should at least contain the number of grams recommended by the Food and Nutrition Board, coupled with an adequate calorie intake.

These protein requirements will also have to be increased in certain conditions, such as during recovery from an operation or in any medical situation involving the need for tissue growth. It is also true that a muscle-building program will require an increase in protein to support the growth.

The protein must be good quality protein. By that I mean it must provide an adequate amount of complete protein, which contains sufficient amounts of all the essential amino acids. These are the amino acids your own body cannot manufacture in sufficient quantity to support body functions. Your body can manufacture many amino acids from other amino acids, and even by forming new amino acids, but it must obtain the essential amino acids it cannot make from your diet. That is why foods that contain complete protein are so important to your diet. These are the meat and dairy groups of foods. The right combination of vegetables may also provide the needed essential amino acids, but being sure to get the right combination is sometimes difficult. The combination of mature bean seeds and corn in sufficient amounts can provide what is needed.

Fats, Vitamins, and Minerals

Only a small amount of polyunsaturated fatty acid, linoleic acid, seems to be essential to body functions. It is wise to limit your saturated fat to no more than a third of your total fat intake.

It is clear that if you are going to limit your fat intake, a major portion of your diet should be from carbohydrates. These are from the fruits, vegetables and cereals in your diet. Your limits on carbohydrates should be determined by your calorie requirements.

You may be wondering how many vitamins and minerals you might need. Solid research studies have shown that even with calorie-restricted diets you cannot improve your nutrition by taking excessive amounts of vitamins and minerals. You do need the recommended daily dietary allowances (RDA). If you are following a regimen that doesn't provide these, you are on the wrong diet. It follows that a weight-losing diet is suspect if it must be supplemented with vitamins and minerals to avoid deficiencies. Usually it is a diet that leads to undernutrition. The two exceptions to this are that women in the childbearing years may need extra iron, and most women—perhaps some men too—need more calcium than is currently provided for by the RDA values. You shouldn't need a bottle of pills as part of your diet.

Food and Nutrition Board, National Academy of Sciences - National Research Council
Recommended Daily Dietary Allowances,[a] Part I: Protein and Minerals (Revised 1980)
Designed for the maintenance of good nutrition of practically all healthy people in the U.S.A.

	Age (years)	Weight (kg)	Weight (lb)	Height (cm)	Height (in)	Protein (g)	Minerals Calcium (mg)	Phosphorus (mg)	Magnesium (mg)	Iron (mg)	Zinc (mg)	Iodine (µg)
Infants	0.0-0.5	6	13	60	24	kg x 2.2	360	240	50	10	3	40
	0.5-1.0	9	20	71	28	kg x 2.0	540	360	70	15	5	50
Children	1-3	13	29	90	35	23	800	800	150	15	10	70
	4-6	20	44	112	44	30	800	800	200	10	10	90
	7-10	28	62	132	52	34	800	800	250	10	10	120
Males	11-14	45	99	157	62	45	1200	1200	350	18	15	150
	15-18	66	145	176	69	56	1200	1200	400	18	15	150
	19-22	70	154	177	70	56	800	800	350	10	15	150
	23-50	70	154	178	70	56	800	800	350	10	15	150
	51+	70	154	178	70	56	800	800	350	10	15	150
Females	11-14	46	101	157	62	46	1200	1200	300	18	15	150
	15-18	55	120	163	64	46	1200	1200	300	18	15	150
	19-22	55	120	163	64	44	800	800	300	18	15	150
	23-50	55	120	163	64	44	800	800	300	18	15	150
	51+	55	120	163	64	44	800	800	300	10	15	150
Pregnant						+30	+400	+400	+150	b	+5	+25
Lactating						+20	+400	+400	+150	b	+10	+50

a The allowances are intended to provide for individual variations among most normal persons as they live in the United States under usual environmental stresses. Diets should be based on a variety of common foods in order to provide other nutrients for which human requirements have been less well defined.

b The increased requirement during pregnancy cannot be met by the iron content of habitual American diets nor by the existing iron stores of many women; therefore the use of 30-60 mg of supplemental iron is recommended. Iron needs during lactation are not substantially different from those of nonpregnant women, but continued supplementation of the mother for 2-3 months after parturition is advisable in order to replenish stores depleted by pregnancy.

Food and Nutrition Board, National Academy of Sciences - National Research Council
Recommended Daily Dietary Allowances, Part II: Vitamins (Revised 1980)
Designed for the maintenance of good nutrition of practically all healthy people in the U.S.A.

	Age (years)	Weight (kg)	Weight (lb)	Height (cm)	Height (in)	Fat-Soluble vitamins A (μg RE)c	D (μg)d	E (mg a-TE)e	Water-Soluble vitamins C (mg)	Thiamin (mg)	Riboflavin (mg)	Niacin (mg NE)f	B-6 (mg)	Folacing (μg)	B-12 (μg)
Infants	0.0-0.5	6	13	60	24	420	10	3	35	0.3	0.4	6	0.3	30	0.5h
	0.5-1.0	9	20	71	28	400	10	4	35	0.5	0.6	8	0.6	45	1.5
Children	1-3	13	29	90	35	400	10	5	45	0.7	0.8	9	0.9	100	2.0
	4-6	20	44	112	44	500	10	6	45	0.9	1.0	11	1.3	200	2.5
	7-10	28	62	132	52	700	10	7	45	1.2	1.4	16	1.6	300	3.0
Males	11-14	45	99	157	62	1000	10	8	50	1.4	1.6	18	1.8	400	3.0
	15-18	66	145	176	69	1000	10	10	60	1.4	1.7	18	2.0	400	3.0
	19-22	70	154	177	70	1000	7.5	10	60	1.5	1.7	19	2.2	400	3.0
	23-50	70	154	178	70	1000	5	10	60	1.4	1.6	18	2.2	400	3.0
	51+	70	154	178	70	1000	5	10	60	1.2	1.4	16	2.2	400	3.0
Females	11-14	46	101	157	62	800	10	8	50	1.1	1.3	15	1.8	400	3.0
	15-18	55	120	163	64	800	10	8	60	1.1	1.3	14	2.0	400	3.0
	19-22	55	120	163	64	800	7.5	8	60	1.1	1.3	14	2.0	400	3.0
	23-50	55	120	163	64	800	5	8	60	1.0	1.2	13	2.0	400	3.0
	51+	55	120	163	64	800	5	8	60	1.0	1.2	13	2.0	400	3.0
Pregnant						+200	+5	+2	+20	+0.4	+0.3	+2	+0.6	+400	+1.0
Lactating						+400	+5	+3	+40	+0.5	+0.5	+5	+0.5	+100	+1.0

c Retinol equivalents. 1 retinol equivalent = 1 μg retinol or 6 μg β carotene.

d As cholecalciferol. 10 μg cholecalciferol = 400 IU of vitamin D.

e a-tocopherol equivalents. 1 mg d-a tocopherol = 1 a-TE.

f 1 NE (niacin equivalent) is equal to 1 mg of niacin or 60 mg of dietary tryptophan.

g The folacin allowances refer to dietary sources as determined by Lactobacillus casei assay after treatment with enzymes (conjugases) to make polyglutamyl forms of the vitamin available to the test organism.

h The recommended dietary allowance for vitamin B-12 in infants is based on average concentration of the vitamin in human milk. The allowances after weaning are based on energy intake (as recommended by the American Academy of Pediatrics) and consideration of other factors, such as intestinal absorption.

Summary 9

1. Calorie requirements can be calculated by measuring your oxygen consumption at rest. You use 4.825 calories for each liter of oxygen you use.
2. Your near-basal calorie requirement equals 30.72 calories a day per kilogram (2.2 pounds) of your fat-free body weight.
3. Normally your brain uses only glucose for energy and it uses 125 grams a day, which is 500 calories.
4. Loss of fat-free body tissue, such as muscles, decreases the number of calories your body can use.
5. If you increase your calorie intake after losing fat-free body tissues that uses calories, you may increase your body fat stores.
6. Many illnesses increase metabolism and increase the loss of heat through the skin.
7. Fifteen percent of your calories should come from complete protein, not more than 30 percent from fat and the rest from carbohydrates.
8. Limit your saturated fat to no more than one-third of your total fat intake and 10 percent of your total calorie intake.
9. You must have at least 125 grams of carbohydrate to meet the brain's requirements for 500 calories a day from glucose.
10. Your diet should be sufficiently balanced with a variety of foods to meet the recommended daily dietary allowance (RDA) for vitamins and minerals.

Chapter 10

Diet Games People Play

In the United States alone, there are probably at least 40 million people on a diet to lose weight. A Nielsen survey reported that 56 percent of women between 25 and 34 years of age were dieting to lose weight. It's not just women. Men are equally as concerned about their weight. It is a myth that men do not want to look good; and right now, looking good means looking lean. So, a vast number of people are playing the diet game. In some instances dieting is really the right thing to do, but in others it leads to undernutrition, with its complications of fatigue and loss of vim, vigor and vitality. A bad diet can take the zest out of living.

Some people have immediate adverse effects from even rather sensible approaches to limiting calorie intake. Sudden changes in dietary habits are not always well tolerated. This lady's letter is an example.

DEAR DR. LAMB: Can you help me lose weight? I am 33 years old and the mother of four. I'm in good health except I weigh 150 pounds and would like to weigh between 130 and 135 pounds. I go to aerobics class three times a week. This makes me feel good, but when I put myself on a diet to lose weight, I get extremely bad headaches. I become weak and have pains in my stomach. The headaches are the worse of the problem and cannot be relieved by aspirin or Tylenol. They can last anywhere from three days to almost two weeks.

This puzzles me because the diet I use is what I call a common sense diet, simply eating smaller portions, lots of vegetables, boiled beef and chicken and avoiding desserts, junk food and colas. The headaches are relieved when I return to my old eating habits, eating anything I want.

Pounds of What?

The number of people playing the diet game has resulted in one popular diet after another. Each claims to be the *real answer* to eliminating those unwanted pounds. Most of these diets range from bad to very bad. A good many depend upon literally fooling the public. P.T. Barnum could have taken lessons from some of these hucksters. For a number of years, you haven't been able to pick up a newspaper or magazine without having your intelligence insulted with ads that claimed that you could lose 10 pounds a week, and go on to lose 20, 30 or even 50 pounds without being hungry. These ads were careful never to say you would lose 10 pounds of body fat in one week. Losing pounds, and losing body fat are not the same thing. Most of those diets that actually did result in loss of pounds were eliminating body water, not pounds of body fat. The other source of the great weight loss was emptying out the intestinal tract, on a diet that provided no residue. These temporary weight losses did nothing for people, other than make them think that at last they had found the secret. A lot of these diets were based on ignorance, some on fraud, and others on both.

Calories Don't Count

The first really heavily marketed diet plan was Dr. Herman Taller's diet, popularized in his book, *Calories Don't Count*, published in 1961. Taller deserves credit, or blame, for really popularizing low-carbohydrate, high-protein diets. Never mind that he got caught up in the legal ramifications of selling safflower capsules with his diet. Knowing what you do about your calorie balance system, and its relationship to the basic Law of Conservation of Energy, you can appreciate that claiming calories don't count is utterly ridiculous. There is no way that calories don't count. None of the diet gurus have found a way to destroy energy, and that includes calories of energy. Energy is neither created nor destroyed. These low-carbohydrate, high-protein diets rely on two fundamental facts. First, if you limit carbohydrates, your kidneys will eliminate sodium. It takes water to eliminate the sodium, so on the first day of little or no carbohydrates, a person may lose several pounds. Pounds of what? Water, not fat! The second fact is that many high-protein foods are really low-calorie foods, and often such a diet is low in calories. Any diet that decreases your calories enough is bound to cause you to have a negative calorie balance, and result in your weight loss.

Another helpful feature of low-carbohydrate diets, and many other low-calorie diets, is that within the first few days the individual's hunger abates. He is no longer ravenous. That is related to basic chemical changes in the body. This was also noted in the young Minnesota men who consumed 1,570 calories a day, and their diet included 300 grams of carbohydrate a day.

The Diet Revolution

The second great wave of the low-carbohydrate diet was *Dr. Atkins' Diet Revolution*, which recycled many of Taller's original claims. It was dressed up with some nice recipes, and the first few days were "no-carbohydrate days." You could eat all you wanted, as long as you didn't eat carbohydrates initially, or very many carbohydrates thereafter. The Atkins diet popularized ketones. Ketones are incompletely utilized fats that are eliminated in the urine. In medical situations, they occur in those diabetics who are out of control and about to go into diabetic acidosis, which can lead to coma. This happens in diabetics because their lack of insulin means they can't burn glucose, so they burn fat. In a way, the lack of insulin, and inability to metabolize glucose, has forced them into a low-carbohydrate system. The test to tell if you had restricted your carbohydrates adequately was to measure the ketones in the urine. Dr. Atkins had the people playing the diet game, catching samples of their urine, and testing it with a little paper tape to see if it changed color or not. If it had not been so pathetic, it would have been hilarious.

The American Medical Association did not think *Dr. Atkins' Diet Revolution* was hilarious. It was the first of the diet books that really reaped a bonanza for the publisher and the author. It alerted many book publishers to the potential profit that could be had from a diet book that promised quick and easy weight loss without pain and suffering. The Council on Foods and Nutrition of the American Medical Association, composed of some of the leading authorities on nutrition, issued a formal statement on the Atkins' diet. Part of what they said is as follows:

The "diet revolution" is neither new nor revolutionary. It is a variant of the familiar low carbohydrate diet that has been promulgated for years. It was first introduced about 100 years ago by an English surgeon. More recently it has reappeared with only slight variations as the "Air Force Diet" in 1960; the diet advocated by Dr. Herman Taller in *Calories Don't Count* in 1961; the *Drinking Man's Diet* in 1964; and Dr. Stillman's *Quick Weight Loss Diet* in 1967.

The rationale advanced to justify the diet is, for the most part, without scientific merit.

The Council was particularly disturbed about the high intake of saturated fat and cholesterol that could result from the Atkins diet because they considered it potentially dangerous to health in terms of causing heart attacks. The highly successful promotion of the book to the public and its quick indiscriminate acceptance motivated the Council on Foods and Nutrition to take this unusual step to safeguard the public's health.

At the time of the frenzy over the Atkins diet, I was a guest on a TV talk show in Houston, Texas, which included Roberta Peters. Like many people who are caught up in the enthusiasm of a new idea, Roberta Peters claimed to have been on the Atkins diet. She glowed over how good she felt on the diet. I calmly told her that I had tried the diet too, and I had felt just awful, that it caused me to have a headache, to feel weak and have a tendency to faint. I will always remember her expression of near shock when she realized that I had actually tried the diet. I tried it so I would know firsthand what effects it would have on people. Then the discussion began in earnest. I asked her point blank if she had ketosis. She evaded the question, so I pressed on to ask her if she had tested her urine. She said she had not. Further discussion revealed that she had not actually eliminated her carbohydrates entirely, as one was supposed to do at the start of the diet. That meant the reason she had felt so good was that she had not been adequately deprived of carbohydrate, so, in fact, had never really been on the Atkins diet. Initially, the person who followed the diet exactly as recommended would lose a lot of salt and water. That salt and water loss would immediately result in fatigue, and a tendency to faint on standing.

Water loss is not fat loss. It can be brought about by many different things. One is space flight. I remember talking to astronaut Ed White, the first man to walk in space, about his experience. He told me that he lost nine pounds during space flight and regained it all the first night back on earth. Weightlessness will do that. Bed rest will do it, too. If your body is properly hydrated, and you stay in bed, you may lose five pounds of weight the first day and not lose an ounce of body fat. My colleagues and I studied many young healthy men at bed rest, in an effort to find out what to expect from space flight. When you get out of bed, or return from space flight, you will quickly regain your lost water. Your body needs that water. If you dehydrate your body, it is like dehydrating your plants. Who wants to have a wilted body?

Increased Risk of Heart Disease and Cancer

The low-carbohydrate, high-protein diets may cause another problem, loading your body with fat and cholesterol. That is particularly true if you are told you can eat anything you like except carbohydrates. The high-fat diets that result are often high in saturated fat, which can greatly increase the cholesterol level in some people. This is very undesirable since it can cause fatty-cholesterol deposits in your arteries and increase your risk of having a heart attack or a stroke. Since milk contains carbohydrates, such diets also restrict milk, and cause a calcium deficiency that can contribute to dissolving bones—osteoporosis.

Can you lose weight on these diets? Yes. *You can lose weight and harm your health.* Certainly, you can't stay on such bad diets indefinitely. The goal in a proper diet is to help the person lose the pounds of body fat that need to be eliminated, without harming his or her health. The latter part is the real trick. After all, if you were just concerned about losing weight, why not get a good case of advanced tuberculosis or cancer? You can lose weight that way too.

That points up another problem with such diets. Many low-carbohydrate, high-protein diets are high-fat diets. High-fat diets may increase a person's risk of both colon cancer and breast cancer. I doubt using such a diet for a few weeks is going to do this. But, clearly, that is a risk one should not take by following such diets on a long-term basis.

The Water Diet

The Stillman diet popularized in *The Doctor's Quick Weight Loss Diet*, which the American Medical Association's Council on Foods and Nutrition cited, isn't really much different. Like the Atkins diet, it eliminates carbohydrates and advocates eating high-protein foods. The fact that it incorporates drinking at least eight glasses of water a day, plus coffee, tea and diet sodas, has caused it to be dubbed the water diet. You can pass this one up, too. It is grossly deficient in needed vitamins and minerals.

Some people have the idea that a liquid diet is the answer to losing weight. This woman's letter is an example.

> DEAR DR. LAMB: Is there a fast way to lose 20 pounds of fat? I am in my early 50s and not so active, therefore the fat wants to stay with me. I'm not a big eater and I would like to know if I just drink juices and liquids, will that bring the weight down fast? I just hate myself with all this fat. I cannot do a lot of exercising because of bronchitis and arthritis and a pinched nerve in the neck. But I need to lose weight fast and bad.

There is nothing magic about liquids other than the fact they provide no bulk and the colon will be empty rather soon. That provides some apparent weight loss, but not the pounds of fat this lady is so anxious to lose. The only other reason a liquid diet will cause weight loss is that it may not provide many calories. Whenever you grossly limit the calorie intake, whether it is with a "water diet," a low-carbohydrate, high-protein diet, or some other diet, you will be in negative calorie balance and start the process of losing body weight, hopefully fat.

Why Not Starve?

With all the demand for quick weight loss, there were those who even recommended eating nothing at all. The changes that occur when you don't eat anything explains a lot about all those bad diets you have heard about, or tried. It also gives you some vital information about when you should eat, and what you should eat. If you don't eat anything, your body must run on the energy already stored as fat or energy used in forming body tissues. Your body will use amino acids from protein, glucose and fat.

The problem is, your body doesn't have a very large glycogen store—the source for glucose—or a large store of amino acids. Your liver only stores about 70 grams of glycogen. There are only about 200 grams of muscle glycogen, and that is not readily available for other cells. There are another 20 grams of glucose in your circulating blood. Even counting the muscle glycogen, that accounts for a total of only

1,160 calories. That is not enough to meet the near-basal calorie requirements for even 24 hours.

The glycogen in your liver is the important source of glucose to maintain your blood level and to provide needed glucose for your brain. Remember, the brain needs 125 grams of glucose for each 24 hours. It is not surprising, then, that the liver glycogen is depleted within 18 to 24 hours after you quit using carbohydrates. Does your brain suffer? Probably. It is sustained by another mechanism. Your liver starts breaking down your amino acids and converting them into glucose, a process called gluconeogenesis, which means the birth of new glucose. The problem with that protective measure is that it rapidly depletes the body protein. Forming glucose from amino acids explains why you will lose a lot of body protein at the onset of a total fast. That should also be a good lesson for people who like to fast one day a week. That initial day of fasting is when you lose the most body protein. Remember that the lost body protein comes from your metabolically-active tissue, and you need it to keep your near-basal energy requirements at a healthy high level. When you lose metabolically-active tissue, you need to limit your calories more after weight loss because your body uses fewer calories.

This process continues for about two to three days. The body is adjusting and switching over to use your major calorie store, your body fat. As it becomes dependent upon burning fat, it releases ketones. The brain is able to switch over and burn ketones for energy instead of glucose, otherwise no one would survive more than the initial day or two of a total fast. After this switch, the body will stop using so much protein, and will use mostly fat as a source of energy, as long as the fast continues, or until the fat stores are depleted. What happens then? You will die. Your body will be forced again to start using its protein as an energy source. Life does not last long after you start depleting your body protein in the latter stages of a prolonged fast.

It is important to realize that after an overnight fast, you will already have depleted about 75 percent of the glycogen in your liver. Your body will have switched over to the starving state, rather than the just-fed state. Your brain will have used all that glucose while you have been sleeping. Your liver has already started mobilizing protein to be converted to glucose. If you want to save your body protein, you must eat breakfast. Moreover, you should include some available carbohydrate in your meals. Your liver and your brain are waiting for it. You need to recharge your liver's glycogen supply to protect your protein. It follows that cereals and fruit are important items for that first meal of the day.

Cowhides and Hoofs

It was soon discovered that one way to minimize the protein loss from starvation was to provide as much protein as the body could break down, so it wouldn't burn the body protein. In the wake of these discoveries, the liquid protein diets were born. Again, people lost weight and were not hungry. But it doesn't pay to abuse your body, and soon the toll of the liquid protein diets became apparent. One of these, the *Last Chance Diet*, consisted of little more than a few ounces of liquid protein. Soon, people who had been subsisting on these starvation diets died. In quick succession, there were 16 deaths, followed by more, which brought in the U.S. Food and Drug Administration (FDA) to investigate. The FDA and the Centers for Disease Control (CDC) soon reported that there were at least 50 brand names of liquid protein products and that they consisted of solutions made from cowhides, collagen and gelatin, with a little saccharin and artificial flavoring. The protein used in these formulas was not complete protein, which led to a progressive protein deficiency. The deaths were often caused by a fatal irregularity of the heart, and the heart muscle itself showed the changes characteristic of starvation. Such low-calorie diets can lead to a loss of potassium, along with other changes, which can cause heart irregularities.

The deaths that occurred in patients on the *Last Chance Diet* led to some revised thinking on the part of those interested in using protein-only-diets that would spare the body's protein. The next step was to provide better protein—complete protein that contained all the essential amino acids as found in real meat and other sources of high quality protein, rather than cowhides and hoofs. The diet was proposed by investigators from the Department of Nutrition and Food Science, Massachusetts Institute of Technology, Cambridge, and Harvard Medical School, Boston. This creation was called the "Protein-Sparing Modified Fast Diet," and provided between 400 and 600 calories of energy, consisting of good quality protein and little else. Of course, the patients lost weight, as people on severe calorie-restricted diets do.

Again, eliminating carbohydrates was a central concept of the diet. The weight loss was directly related to the negative calorie balance used in such a program.

Although a lot of emphasis was placed on eliminating carbohydrates, some skeptics asked out loud if it wasn't still true that calories did count, and would you get the same results from diets that contained the same number of calories, but also contained carbohydrate. Dr. Philip Felig and colleagues at Yale University School of Medicine then tested obese individuals with a 400-calorie protein diet, and also a 400-calorie diet that had 50 percent of its calories from carbohydrate and 50 percent from protein. They found that the mixed diet of 50 percent carbohydrate was just as effective as the plain protein diet in sparing the body's protein. Since the purpose of the Protein-Sparing Modified Fast Diet was to spare the body protein, it clearly offered no advantages, and nothing unique, except for a few little things. The pure protein diet resulted in a higher level of ketone bodies, it caused the body to lose more sodium and water and caused the subjects to be more prone to fainting than patients on the mixed diet. It also affected the body's level of norepinephrine, part of the body's sympathetic nervous system function. Most people could do very well without these little extras caused by eliminating carbohydrates entirely.

Today, the high-protein low-carbohydrate modified fast programs are being used again, often by hospitals, and they are being done under doctors' supervision. Two of these are Optifast and Medifast. The Optifast formula provides five packages that contain 84 calories each, of which 14 grams are protein, 6 grams are carbohydrate and 0.4 grams are fat. The Medifast program provides five packets of 94 calories each and each package contains 14 grams of protein, 8 grams of carbohydrate and 0.8 grams of fat and 0.4 grams of dietary fiber. Both are spiked with the Recommended Dietary Allowances of vitamins and minerals.

These programs are for the markedly obese who have life threatening conditions associated with their obesity. There are people who become so obese or respond so adversely to their obesity in terms of blood pressure and high total cholesterol levels that it is important to induce a rapid weight loss. But most obese people do not require such heroic efforts. These new high-protein, modified fasts are not greatly different from diets that have not had a good track record in terms of keeping excess weight off and in terms of their effects on health. The jury is still out on this current practice.

High on Carbohydrates

After finding out all those drawbacks to the low-carbohydrate diets, why not reverse directions and use lots of carbohydrates? Whether it was intended to do that or not, that is essentially what the popular Beverly Hills Diet proposed. Judy Mazel's *The Beverly Hills Diet* book was the number-one best-seller for months. Only seven percent of the calories in the Beverly Hills Diet is from protein, far below the RDA for protein intake. Just 12 percent of its calories are fat, and the rest is carbohydrate. Judy Mazel was once an overweight woman who lost weight by dieting. She is not the first popular diet guru to take that path to success. Unfortunately, her concepts of nutrition are not based on known scientific facts. Dr. Arthur H. Hayes, Jr., Commissioner for the Food and Drug Administration when Mazel's diet was popularized, was quoted from an interview as saying, "The Beverly Hills diet is based on the ludicrous idea that certain combinations of foods clog your stomach's enzyme system and prevent food from being digested. As a result, food turns into fat. Mazel says that 'fruits should be eaten alone or else they get trapped by other foods in your stomach.' Along the same lines, protein should only be eaten with other proteins, etc. Mazel's misconceptions about enzymes, the biological catalysts involved in the digestive process, could set molecular biology back twenty years."

He went on to say, "However, the diet is grossly inadequate nutritionally and may be dangerous. It can lead to potassium deficiency which could cause potentially fatal abnormal heart rhythms. People on this diet have become seriously ill due to diarrhea and dehydration. Fortunately, to the best of our knowledge, the diet hasn't killed anyone yet. *The Beverly Hills Diet* is full of misinformation so strange that it would be funny, except that so many people seem to believe it. Our favorite misconception is Mazel's claim that potatoes, if eaten with meat, ferment into vodka in your stomach and make you intoxicated."

A Little Malabsorption

It seems the only limitation on diet games people play is the imagination of the players. After looking for the magic combination of foods that would defy the laws of energy, along came the approach of preventing absorption of calories. It is quite true that before a calorie counts, it has to get into the system. That means it has to be digested, and absorbed through the intestinal wall into the bloodstream. Doctors are very familiar with patients who have malabsorption diseases. These are patients with diseases of the pancreas or intestines that prevent them from absorbing what they eat. Most of these patients have real problems, including diarrhea, gaseous distension, abdominal cramps, and vitamin and mineral deficiencies. If you cannot digest a food, it is fermented in the intestine by bacteria, and causes many such problems. A good simple example is lactose intolerance. People who don't have enough of the lactase enzyme to digest lactose sugar in milk have such symptoms.

But P.T. Barnum would have been proud of the marketing associated with the selling of the starch blockers. What did they do? They caused a form of malabsorption disease. By preventing the normal digestion and absorption of starch, the starch was available for fermentation and causing the symptoms of malabsorption. Will they cause you to lose weight? Of course they will. And they are better than tuberculosis or cancer, and perhaps you won't mind the gas and abdominal pain or the loss of nutrients that malabsorption may cause. But the FDA investigated, and your opportunity to lose weight with a little case of malabsorption with that method was ended.

Then there is the fiber pill called glucomannan. What is glucomannan? It is a hydrophilic hemicellulose from the konjac root from Japan. The term hydrophilic hemicellulose means it is a fiber that absorbs water—a bulking agent. In many respects, it is like a lot of the bulk laxatives available, which are also hydrophilic cellulose products that cannot be digested by humans. Will glucomannan work? Yes, if you use bulk to induce distention of your digestive tract, and that helps you curb your appetite, it could help you eat less. That means you are back to the original premise. If you consume and absorb fewer calories than your body uses, regardless of how you get youself to do this, you will be in negative caloric balance, and eventually you will lose weight.

Do It Yourself Diets

People often design some of the worst diet plans on their own with-

out any help from anybody, as my regular mail reveals. Here is one of
the really bad examples.

> DEAR DR. LAMB: I am very worried about my friend. She is 37
> years old and has been dieting for 13 months. I would guess she has lost
> about 50 pounds. She eats only broccoli, cauliflower, carrots and cel-
> ery. She was occasionally adding milk products to her diet, but has
> stopped for fear of gaining weight. She exercises every night, and I'm
> afraid that since she has gotten rid of all her fat, that she is destroying
> muscle.
> Should I be concerned? Is she really doing this right? I'm very proud
> of what she has accomplished, but I'm just afraid she may cause prob-
> lems for herself. Is a vegetable-only diet good for you after this amount
> of time?

While 50 pounds in 13 months is less than a pound a week, the
diet as described is completely unsatisfactory. One can balance a
vegetable, fruit and cereal diet that meets most of the requirements,
but such diets are quite different than the diet that is described here.
I would be greatly concerned about undernutrition, calcium deficiencies, protein deficiencies, iron deficiencies and vitamin deficiencies, just to mention a few of the things that are wrong. Again,
you can lose weight on almost any diet that sufficiently decreases
the calorie intake, even by fasting, but the real goal is to lose unhealthy pounds of fat, if you are not programmed to need that fat,
while not damaging your health, and to develop dietary patterns that
will be good for you and your weight for the rest of your life. Diets
that tear down your energy-producing tissues do not meet those
standards.

Summary 10

1. The large weight loss in the first few days of low-calorie, low-
   carbohydrate diets is mostly loss of the body's normal water content and emptying of the colon—not loss of fat.
2. No-carbohydrate or very-low-carbohydrate diets that result in a
   marked loss of normal body water lead to fatigue, faintness on
   standing and often cause a headache.
3. Some low-carbohydrate high-protein diets that advocate lots of
   foods containing saturated fats may significantly increase the total

cholesterol level and may contribute to a heart attack.

4. Very-low-carbohydrate diets restrict milk because of its lactose sugar. This leads to calcium deficiency which may contribute to osteoporosis.

5. Drinking lots of water or fluids will not affect your fat stores. The extra water is simply eliminated through your kidneys.

6. The liver glycogen which supplies needed glucose for your brain is depleted with 18 to 24 hours after you stop using carbohydrates.

7. When carbohydrates are not available, the liver converts amino acids from proteins into glucose.

8. The conversion of amino acids to glucose results in loss of body protein the first two days of a fast.

9. During the first few days of a fast, your body is switching over to use fat for energy. Incompletely used fat produces ketones—the same thing diabetics in danger of diabetic coma produce.

10. Low-calorie high-protein diets have resulted in a series of cardiac deaths from the loss of important body minerals such as potassium and starvation degeneration of the heart muscle.

Chapter 11

Planning Your Diet

There are many people who are overweight simply because they eat too much high-calorie food. The amount of energy they consume is more than their metabolic furnace can process, so the extra calories must be stored as fat deposits. These people can improve their health, and their appearance, by decreasing their caloric intake. In many instances, this can be done by simply switching to different eating patterns. The calorie balancing mechanism will adjust a person's weight gradually to its proper level. A good example from the animal world is the ordinary laboratory rat. If fed a regular rat diet, not excessively rich in calories, it will not get fat, even if allowed to eat all it wants. That is fairly typical of the animal world. If you leave animals in their natural environment, eating the foods that their bodies were designed through the ages to consume, they usually do not become excessively overweight. The exception is the animal that needs to put on lots of fat for the time when food will not be available, such as a bear preparing for hibernation. If the rat's regular diet is changed to foods rich in calories, or one adds snacks high in fat and sweets, the rat will get fat. He eats about the same amount, but the food contains a lot more calories. Something like that has happened to humans. Under normal circumstances, early man ate foods that were not calorie-rich. When he foraged or gathered grains, there was not a lot of opportunity to consume calorie-rich foods. It was not too long ago in history that sugar was unknown. I am not implying that sugar is always bad, but it is a good example of how man has enriched his diet in terms of calories. About the only sweetener available to early man was from honey, and that was in short supply.

The change in the foods available to man is characterized by this person's letter about junk foods.

DEAR DR. LAMB: I need help fast! I believe I am a junk food junky. I always have to be eating sweets or drinking soda. I never eat a proper meal because I just never feel up to it. I don't like very many vegetables and I just like normal American junk food. I need an exercise program to get into and I also need to get a set diet. I seem to eat junk food 24 hours a day. I've tried a lot of exercise programs but nothing seems to fit into my schedule, or I get bored with them very fast.

Junk food is not a very descriptive term, but sweets and sodas do not remotely resemble the type of foods available to our biological ancestors, or even a few hundred years ago. Our biological system does not change that fast in relation to our environment. Humans are very adaptable, but there are limits. The ready availability of calorie-rich foods is one reason why many people today have problems in controlling their weight.

Add refrigeration to the development of a vast array of new high-calorie food products. It became possible to keep lots of high-calorie foods available. Butter didn't get rancid under refrigeration. Ice cream was no longer a dessert reserved for special occasions a few times a year. Eating ice cream became a daily ritual in many households. We have had our food changed, and many of us, just like the rat, have gained weight on calorie-rich foods. Of course mankind also developed a way of life that didn't involve so much work, and that decreased his calorie requirements. With these changes, it is not surprising that many people became overweight from simply consuming too many calories and not using enough calories. There are two approaches to solving this problems; consuming fewer calories and increasing your calorie use, primarily through increased physical activity. The difficulty comes when what is perceived as excess body fat is not actually excess, and is not caused by consuming too many calories.

Why It Is High Or Low

If you need to restrict calories, you will need to follow at least some general guidelines. The diet need not be a rigid ritual. In most cases, unless a medical problem is also involved, simply switching to foods with a low-calorie density, along with a sensible program of physical activity, is adequate.

How do you choose foods that are low in calorie density? You need to be aware of the factors that cause a food to have a lot of calories. The number one offender is fat. Fat provides nine calories per gram, and is the major source of excess calories in most diets. Your first goal should be to eliminate foods that contain lots of fat, and to prepare foods without using fat. Incidentally, many recipes that call for some fat can be used by simply omitting the fat. You would be surprised how often it is really not needed.

The second factor that affects the number of calories in a food is its water content. This is often overlooked, but most of our natural foods, in their unprocessed state, have been watered down. Take lean round steak as an example. Over 70 percent of its actual weight is water. The result is, if you remove all the visible fat, a pound of lean, raw round steak will contain only about 600 calories. That is a lot of meat, which provides a lot of good quality protein, without loading your energy system with excess calories. The same applies to vegetables and fruits. A raw potato is 80 percent water. Raw fish is about 80 percent water. Now, think again about sugar. It contains almost no water, perhaps 0.5 percent of its weight. That is the real reason it contains so many calories. Its two components, glucose and fructose, are found in fruits, vegetables and cereals, which are usually low-calorie foods. Sugar, after all, is prepared by extracting it from natural foods, the sugar beet and sugar cane. Neither the raw sugar beet nor the sugar cane is high in calories, but when you remove all the water and the fiber, what you have left is refined sugar, which is high in calories. It follows that foods that contain lots of sugar are high in calories.

The third factor that will affect whether a food is high or low in calories is bulk. Our ability to refine and process foods has led to removing a lot of the bulk from our diet. That means the refined product contains a lot more calories per gram, or per ounce, than before the bulk was removed. We are really talking about fiber. It is important in terms of providing bulk for your digestive system, but it is also important to provide bulk for appetite satisfaction, while avoiding overloading yourself with calories. Many of our starch foods are processed foods. White flour is a high-calorie food because it contains no fiber, and very little water. It begins to look a lot like sugar in terms of calories, and that is why an overabundance of starch in your diet may result in your consuming more calories than your system can use.

Sometimes, I am tempted to tell a person who is overweight from simply eating too many calories to forget about diets and just eliminate the sweets, the fats and the processed foods that contain a lot of flour. In most cases, the decreased calories per pound of food will mean the person will have diet satisfaction, and will be consuming less calories. Like the laboratory rat that returned to eating foods less rich in calories, his body weight in time will adjust to the level it should be.

There is one other food item that deserves special mention—alcohol. Alcohol is a hydrocarbon, like your other foodstuffs. It is burned by your body to carbon dioxide and water. It has about seven calories per gram. It is almost as bad as fat. Many people are fat because of their alcohol consumption. Alcohol is truly an "empty calorie" food, as it provides no bulk, no vitamins, no minerals, no amino acids, only calories. In addition, it has many adverse effects on cells. Its drug action eliminates will power, which often results in a person eating more food than usual. If not, and it replaces calories of good healthy foods, it may result in malnutrition. Many people are actually unaware that alcohol is a source of calories and others think that alcohol in beer or wine is somehow different. That is why the person who wrote this letter is confused about the calories in Pearl Light.

DEAR DR. LAMB: What is in beer that is fattening? For example, Pearl Light, which has 68 calories. The analysis on the can states: carbohydrates, 2.6 grams, protein, 0.5 grams and fat, 0.0 grams. The calorie count I assume comes from the carbohydrate. What is the ingredient that makes up the carbohydrate, and is this fattening?

Of course the missing ingredient is not carbohydrate but alcohol. And yes, it is fattening.

The Basic Four

To help you organize your own diet at the calorie level you want, let's take a look at the basic food groups, and how to eliminate the calorie-rich foods, but still provide a balanced diet.

The dairy group is essential to your health. These foods are the major source of calcium in your diet. They also provide phosphorus and complete protein. The protein in milk is good quality complete protein. The problem with some foods in the dairy group is their fat content. About half of the calories in ordinary whole milk are from fat. If you use low-fat milk, containing 2% fat, about a third of the calories are still from fat. Milk is not just a protein food. Unless we do something to it, it is really a high-fat food. It also contains a reasonable amount of cholesterol. That also applies to all dairy products made from whole milk, and, of course, butter. But you can use milk products on a calorie-controlled diet without qualms. Use the protein-fortified skim milk products. They contain almost no fat or cholesterol. There will be only about 94 calories in an 8-ounce glass of this milk. When you are cooking you can use it in your recipes rather than whole milk.

You can also use nonfat dry milk powder. It can be reconstituted and used in cooking, rather than protein fortified skim milk.

You can use low-calorie cottage cheese. This cheese is made without adding the creamy covering seen in ordinary cottage cheese. The low-fat cottage cheese has most of the advantages of low-fat milk. Buttermilk is another low-fat dairy product you can use, as a beverage or in cooking.

The meat group is often avoided because people think all meat is high in fat and cholesterol. Actually, meat can be your friend in providing good quality complete protein, without overloading your calorie balance. When choosing red meats, you need to select cuts that are as lean as possible without evidence of marbling. Remove all the visible fat before cooking. Round steak, or a roast of round, is a good choice. As I mentioned before, a whole pound of raw round steak, with all the fat removed, will contain only about 600 calories. It is wise to avoid cuts that contain lots of fat.

Poultry can be a low-calorie food. All you need to do is select a relatively lean bird, remove the skin and all the visible fat. The breast of chicken or turkey, with the skin removed before cooking, is an excellent source of complete protein and is very low in fat. The dark meat contains a little more fat, but is quite acceptable if skinned before cooking.

Fish is another food that is a low-calorie item. There are fish that are lean and other fish that contain quite a few calories because of their fat content. But since 80 percent of their weight is water, most fish are relatively low-calorie items.

The fruit and vegetable group is not a problem, with a few minor exceptions. Most of them are relatively low in calories. Avocados are a high-fat, high-calorie item. If you really ate a lot of bananas, you could consume a lot of calories. But for the most part, fruits and vegetables are low-calorie items. The problem occurs when we add something to them, such as butter on a baked potato, or a calorie-rich salad dressing.

The bread and cereal group is usually low in calories, also, unless you add something to them. A bowl of oatmeal won't contain many calories until you add a couple of teaspoons of sugar and a pitcher of cream. You do need to be careful about baked goods. The usual breads are relatively low in calories, but sweet rolls, and many commercially baked products, contain a lot of fat as well as sugar. Most people think of meat when they think of fat, but baked goods are often a hidden source of a lot of fat.

Bake, Boil Or Broil

There is one other aspect of calories in your food that you need to consider, how the food is prepared. It is important to bake, boil or broil, and not fry. A lot of fat is added in some methods of food preparation. The breading and frying of meats and vegetables adds an enormous number of calories of fat. This 14-year-old girl has already learned that food preparation is important.

DEAR DR. LAMB: I'm 14 years old and am trying to learn as much as I can about good nutrition. I know it is very important to your health and I want to be healthy, and when I grow up I want to know how to take good care of my family.

My mom is a good cook but she doesn't know anything about what is good for you and what is bad. She's overweight, too, and I think it is because she eats so many fried foods and fats. She takes vitamins every day and says that will take care of anything she is not getting in her diet.

There may be many reasons why this girl's mother is overweight, but certainly fried food and fats can make it hard to avoid overloading her metabolic furnace. If you want to limit your calorie intake, or need to, you should forget about frying foods.

Is It Balanced?

A good balanced diet should include four servings from the dairy group, four servings from the vegetable and fruit group, four servings from the bread and cereal group and two servings from the meat group. You can remember this as the 4,4,4,2 rule. Some people would say you needed only two servings from the dairy group, but you really need four servings to ensure an adequate amount of calcium, and that ensures a good intake of complete protein, too. Your fruit and vegetable group should include an adequate source of vitamin C, such as orange juice or grapefruit juice, or fresh oranges or grapefruit.

I am including a list of foods that you can use as a basis for constructing your own diet. I am including it only because I know that many people do like to have a plan to follow. This can be the basis for a diet that is about 1,300 calories and will be a balanced diet. Since most people should be consuming more calories than this, you can simply increase the number of servings, the size of servings, or add other low-calorie foods not on the list. You will find that you can also use this diet plan for a low-fat, low-cholesterol diet.

Below is an example of the kind of menu you could construct from this list. Notice it provides about 1,300 calories and more than 70 grams of good quality protein from the dairy and meat group.

No one should be on a diet that provides fewer calories than this except under a doctor's supervision. *Usually, a person is better off to increase his exercise, rather than to decrease his calorie intake below the level provided for in this diet.* Since the diet is planned using the four basic food groups, it provides a balanced diet. If you want to increase your calorie intake, you don't need to change your diet drastically. You can simply add items of your choice to it. One of the bad features of many diets is that they are so different from normal eating habits that people do not like to stay on them, or they are not intended to be followed after you lose weight. As a result, a person tends to return to former habits that contributed to being overweight in the first place. One of the important lessons of the weighting game is that you have to construct a pattern of calorie intake and expenditure that you can live with the rest of your life. After a short-term diet, most people regain any weight they have lost. As soon as you are off the diet, your body will seek its normal range of weight. Over 90 percent of people playing the diet game regain everything they lost. Those who decreased their

List A: Vitamin C

One of these items:	calories
1 8-oz glass of orange juice	110
1 (252 gm) large orange	87
2 (262 gm) small oranges	90
1 8-oz glass of grapefruit juice	90
1 (400 gm) whole grapefruit	80
1 (600 gm) medium grapefruit	116

List B: Dairy

Four of these items:

8-oz protein-fortified skim milk (10 gm protein)	94
8-oz buttermilk (8.8 gm protein)	88
1½ cup dry-curd cottage cheese (37 gm protein)	185
1½ cup 1% fat cottage cheese(42 gm protein)	246
1 cup yogurt, plain, lowfat (12 gm protein)	113

List C: Bread and Cereal

2 slices of bread (1 slice = 1 oz) OR 2 dinner rolls	150

plus one of these items

2-oz 40% Bran Flakes	186
2-oz Corn Flakes	220
2-oz Grape-Nuts Flakes	204
2 cups Wheaties	202
2½ cups Puffed Wheat,	134
2 biscuits (47.2 gm) shredded wheat	166
1 cup oatmeal, cooked	145
1 cup rice, cooked	186

List D: Meat, Poultry, Fish

Two of these items:

3½ oz (100 gm), separable lean, raw, of:

beef (21.6 gm protein)	150
ham, lean class (19.8 gm protein)	135
leg of lamb (19.9 gm protein)	127
liver, beef, calf or hog (19.9 protein)	140
½ chicken breast (95 gm, 16% bone), raw (25.7 gm protein)	160
1 (65 gm) thigh (15 gm protein)	122

3½ oz (100 gm), separable lean, edible portion only, of:

cod (17.6 gm protein)	78
croaker (18.0 gm protein)	96
flounder (16.7 gm protein)	79
haddock (18.3 gm protein)	79
halibut (20.9 gm protein)	100
mullet (19.6 gm protein)	146
ocean perch (18.0 gm protein)	88
sanddabs (16.7 gm protein)	79
sole (16.7 gm protein)	79
1 cup (155 gm) crab, blue, Dungeness, rock or king, cooked, not packed (26.8 gm protein)	144
1 cup lobster, cooked (27.1 gm protein)	138
1 cup oysters, raw, 13-19 medium or 19-31 small (20.2 gm protein)	158
3½ oz (100 gm) shrimp, raw, edible portion (18.1 gm protein)	91

List E: Fruits and Vegetables

Four of these items:	calories
1 cup asparagus, cooked, drained	30
1 cup beans, green, yellow or wax, cooked	44
$^2/_3$ cup broccoli, cooked	27
$^2/_3$ cup brussels sprouts, cooked	37
1 cup cabbage, cooked	30
1 cup carrots, cooked	30
1 cup cauliflower, cooked	25
1 cup chard leaves, cooked	32
1 cup collards, cooked	55
$3^1/_2$ oz (100 gm) cress, garden, raw	32
1 (175 gm) cucumber, small	25
1 cup (105 gm) cucumber, sliced	16
1 cup dandelion greens, cooked	60
1 cup eggplant, boiled	38
1 cup endive, cut or broken pieces	10
$3^1/_2$ oz (100 gm) lettuce	15
$^1/_4$ head (wedge) (135 gm) lettuce	18
1 cup mushrooms, raw	20
$^2/_3$ cup mustard greens, cooked	23
1 cup okra, boiled	46
$^1/_2$ cup onions, mature, raw, chopped	33
1 cup onions, green, tops and bulb, chopped	36
$^1/_2$ cup peas, green, cooked	58
1 (200 gm) pepper, immature green, raw	36
1 (135 gm) pickle, dill or sour	15
4 oz (113 gm) pimientos, canned, solids and liquid	31

	calories
$3^1/_2$ oz (100 gm) potatoes, pared, boiled	86
5 oz (143 gm) radishes, edible portion only	23
$^2/_3$ cup spinach cooked	27
$^1/_2$ cup squash	
acorn	55
butternut	68
hubbard	50
winter	63
$3^1/_2$ oz (100 gm) sweet potatoes, boiled in skin	114
7 oz (200 gm) tomato, raw	40
1 cup turnip greens, cooked	30
$3^1/_2$ oz (100 gm) apricot, raw edible portion	51
$^1/_2$ banana, medium size	50
$3^1/_2$ oz (100 gm) muskmelon or cantaloupe, netted	30
$3^1/_2$ oz (100 gm) nectarine, raw, edible portion	64
$3^1/_2$ oz (100 gm) papaya, raw	36
$3^1/_2$ oz (100 gm) peaches, raw, edible portion	38
1 (180 gm) pear, raw	100
6 oz (188 gm) pineapple juice	103
1 cup (155 gm) pineapple, raw, diced	81
1 cup (246 gm) pineapple, canned, water pack	96
1 cup (170 gm) plums, Damson, raw, pitted halves	112
1 cup (185 gm) plums, japanese and hybrid, raw pitted	89
$3^1/_2$ oz (100 gm) strawberries, raw	37

Sample Menu	
Breakfast	
1 grapefruit (600 gm)	116
1 cup oatmeal, cooked	145
1 8-oz glass protein fortified skim milk	94
Calories	**355**
Lunch	
1 8-oz glass protein fortified skim milk	94
$3^1/_2$ oz lettuce	15
$^1/_2$ tomato	20
$^1/_2$ whole chicken breast	160
$^1/_2$ cup green peas cooked	58
1 slice of bread (1 slice = 1 oz)	75
Calories	**422**
Dinner	
1 8-oz glass protein fortified skim milk	94
$1^1/_2$ cup dry curd cottage cheese	185
$^1/_2$ tomato	20
$3^1/_2$ oz flounder	79
1 cup carrots	30
1 cup spinach	27
1 slice of bread (1 slice = 1 oz)	75
Calories	**510**
TOTAL CALORIES	**1287**

active metabolic tissue because of stringent dieting, which used body protein, may actually gain to the point that they weigh more than they did before they started the diet.

What About Vitamins?

Do you need to take vitamins and minerals with this diet? You shouldn't. Since you can plan a balanced diet, you should get all the calcium, iron, vitamins and minerals your system requires. Taking additional vitamins will not help you lose weight or increase your energy level. If your energy level is too low, you need to be sure you do not have a medical problem. It may mean that you are not getting enough calories. This diet is like any other diet, if it doesn't provide enough calories for your daily requirements, you can progressively become a victim of undernutrition.

Vitamins are not a source of energy. They are simply a catalyst to enable your cells to burn your food with oxygen to release its energy. That is where the energy is. You can think of vitamins as the spark plug on an engine. It provides the spark to ignite the combustion of gasoline, but the energy that runs the engine comes from the gasoline. If you do not have enough of the right vitamins, then your metabolic system will be inefficient and you may not burn your foods properly. It is like having dirty spark plugs—they may make it impossible for the engine to fire the gasoline properly. So you do need vitamins and minerals, but they should come from your balanced diet.

People who are not on a balanced diet for any reason, which is true of many people who live alone or are older, do need to take an ordinary preparation that provides the RDA for vitamins. But note carefully, this is only necessary for people who are not on a proper diet. If you need additional vitamins because they are not provided by your diet, you are probably on the wrong diet plan.

Some Reasons for Carbohydrates

It is a good idea to have a major portion of your calorie intake as carbohydrates. The best carbohydrate foods are the more complex ones, but, if your calorie intake will allow it, the pastas, spaghetti and breads are good for you. Carbohydrates provide the energy for your muscles when you initially engage in vigorous physical activity. Champion athletes and their coaches have demonstrated that an adequate intake of carbohydrates can be useful in preparing for endurance events. Since you want to avoid too much fat, and you don't need a lot of extra protein, the best source for additional calories is carbohydrates. For the person engaged in regular vigorous physical activities, that can include sweets. Just remember that most candy also contains a lot of fat, not just sugar. If you like meat and want to increase your calories, there is no reason not to eat more fish, poultry or lean red meats in addition to your other foods. There are no special advantages from increasing your protein rather than your carbohydrate, unless you are in a muscle-building program or have an illness that requires an increase in protein intake.

Remember that your brain uses 125 grams of glucose a day. That means that your diet should include at least this much carbohydrate just to feed your brain. If you were on a low-carbohydrate diet that caused you to form ketones, that would not be true, but I do not recommend such diets. If you don't provide enough carbohydrate for the brain, and for some other purposes, you run the risk that your body will use its own protein to form glucose for your essential needs.

Also, remember that most of your liver glycogen will be depleted by the time you wake up after a night's sleep. You will need to replace that liver glycogen early to avoid using body protein. That is why your breakfast should include a reasonable amount of carbohydrate.

Summary 11

1. Many of the high-calorie foods available today are not the natural fare that was available to our ancestors. Consumption of these foods overloads the metabolic furnace and results in overweight.
2. Fats are the highest calorie source in our foods, providing 9 calories per gram.
3. Water in foods such as vegetables, lean meat, fish and fruit decrease their calories per pound. Foods with little or no water content contain lots of calories—like sugar, honey and flour.
4. Undigestable bulk in food such as fiber decreases the calories per pound, but refined foods, such as sugar, contain lots of calories.
5. Alcohol contains 7 calories per gram and is a frequent cause of excess calorie intake.
6. A balanced diet should include four servings each from the vegetable and fruit group, the bread and cereal group, the dairy group and two servings from the meat group each day—the 4-4-4-2 rule.
7. How food is prepared is a major factor in its calorie content—bake it, boil it or broil it.
8. Vitamins do not provide calories, but they are essential in burning foods in your metabolic furnace to release calories.
9. Carbohydrates are an ideal food for a major portion of the calorie intake in healthy diets. By choosing the complex carbohydrate foods—the fresh fruits and vegetables and the bread and the cereals—you can provide bulk satisfaction without overloading the metabolic furnace.

Chapter 12

Why Exercise Is Essential

How useful is exercise in helping you to lose weight? If it is, which exercises are best to lose weight? Exercise is an important part of any program to eliminate extra body fat. I think it is so important that I always recommend that anyone who decreases calories to lose weight should start an exercise program at the same time if they are not already involved in a reasonable amount of physical activity. Here is an example from one lady on what she accomplished by also using exercise.

DEAR DR. LAMB: I am a 33-year-old woman, 5 feet 1 inch tall and now weigh 131 pounds. A year ago I went to my doctor and she said I had to lose 35 pounds, which I have done. She put me on a bland diet. Since exercise is important I got involved in aerobic dance exercises which really worked. I lost inches in places I never thought I could. My measurements before were: bust, 41½, waist 35, hips 43. My weight was 165 pounds. Now my measurements are 38, 28, 37 and I weigh 131 pounds. I feel great and everyone tells me I look great.

My question to you, Dr. Lamb is, must I stick to the same exercise program or increase it? When I work out now I really don't feel any tension. Does that mean the exercise is not doing any good any more? Do I stay on the same diet?

The exercise undoubtedly played an important part in this woman losing weight and feeling great. She evidently lost less than a pound of weight a week while improving her level of physical fitness. As she increased her exercise capacity, she increased the metabolically

143

active tissue and that will help her avoid regaining the body fat she has lost.

The ease with which she does her workouts today does not mean that the exercise is not doing her any good. That just means that she is now in much better physical condition than she was before she started her program. Her exercise uses calories and turns on her heat-loss mechanism. It is an important part in helping her avoid regaining body fat. And after a year, she has probably set a new level that balances her calories in with her calories out. If she wants to eat more, she can increase her exercise and stay at the same weight.

There are millions of people jogging, running, playing racquetball, attending aerobics classes, lifting weights and working their muscles against the latest exercise machines. This change in our culture has been called the fitness boom. It got a lot of its impetus from the belief that exercise could prevent heart disease. It is important in preventing fatty-cholesterol deposits and the complication of heart attacks. But a lot of these effects are because of the way exercise affects your calorie balance system. You can use exercise to build your fat-free metabolic tissue, and that is good, or you can misuse exercise to tear down your metabolic tissues and reserves, and that is bad. Exercise, like diet, can be friendly or unfriendly to your body. It depends on how you do it. If you use it right, it can be your best aid to achieve you proper weight and to keep it there. Exercise needs to be kept in balance with your nutrition—your calorie intake.

Getting Fat from Inactivity

Exercise literally turns on your metabolic furnace and liberates calories of heat. That is why people sweat when they exercise enough. Dieting shuts down your metabolic furnace and causes you to use less calories. It is not surprising that exercise can make you feel more energetic, while dieting can make you tired.

Lack of exercise can make you fat. Livestock farmers have used this fact for years. That is what a feed lot is all about. If cattle are kept in a very small area, where their activity is limited, and given ample calories of food, they get fat, ready for market. If you allow these small animals to roam the range, despite feeding them all they want, they are going to be much leaner. The ultimate example of this is the "grass-fat" animal from the range, with its tougher muscle fibers from exercise and lean carcass. It is important to restrict an animal's activity to make it fat. The same principle is used in fattening almost all animals. The chicken farmer raises chickens for market in the same way. They are caged in a limited space and their rations are increased. The end result is the fat bird, with tender muscles, ready for market. Some consider them to be tasteless rubber-chicken compared to the free-roaming barnyard bird. The list of animals that are fattened by limiting their activity is endless.

Humans are no different. Inactivity is one of the major causes of obesity in our society of people who are relatively inactive and have a ready access to calorie-rich foods. The end result is an overweight population with soft, underworked muscles that are not fulfilling their metabolic potential. You might say many of them are "ready for market."

Before the age of affluence, people walked because they did not have automobiles. The human body was designed and developed over thousands of years to be active and to walk. Your metabolic system was designed to support a creature who walked, ran and was active. In the past, people often had to perform chores, such as bringing wood into the house, instead of turning up the thermostat. Before telephones, radios and TV, people relied on games for entertainment, and that often meant physical activity.

Exercise Stimulates Heat Release

Look at your energy model and see how exercise fits into the scheme. When your muscles contract, they release heat. In fact, over 75 percent of the calories used in muscular contraction are released as heat. That is a lot like your automobile engine. If your engine has been running a little while, you know better than to put your bare hand on it, or to open the radiator cap. You know it is hot. Only a small amount of the energy released by your automobile engine is transformed into mechanical energy to move your auto down the road. The rest is released as heat, and makes your motor hot. Your muscles do the same thing. They process hydrocarbons from your food, just as your auto engine processes gasoline (hydrocarbon). In both systems, oxygen burns the hydrocarbons to carbon dioxide and water, as the energy in

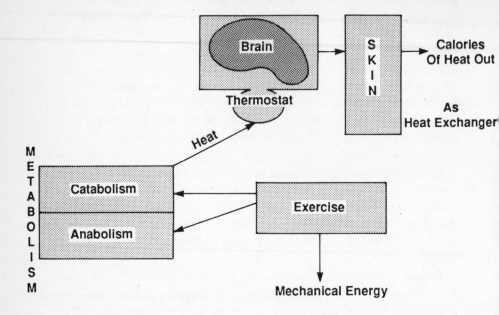

Exercise drives the brain to release calories of heat, to use calories to build (anabolism) and to use some calories for mechanical energy.

the hydrocarbons is released. Your muscles convert less than 25 percent of the energy as mechanical energy to enable you to dance, run or play tennis. The remainder is released as heat.

As you exercise, the heat in your body increases, just like the motor of your auto. Your body temperature rises and your thermostat in your brain senses this. Immediately, your brain turns on the heat loss system to get rid of calories of heat. You can think again of the analogy of your body being a large room with a furnace at one end and an air conditioner at the other, with a thermostat sensing the temperature in the room. As the furnace puts out more heat, the thermostat perceives it and turns on the air conditioner. That is exactly what happens with your body when you exercise. The exercise increases the heat put out by your metabolic furnace. Your thermostat perceives the rise in temperature, and your brain turns on your air conditioner—your skin. Blood flow through the skin increases, so a person who is exercising fairly vigorously will be flushed. That aids in eliminating calories by radiation and convection. As the exercise continues, evaporative cooling is increased by the action of your sweat glands, stimulated through your brain. Finally, as the body is overloaded with excessive heat, dripping sweat follows.

If you are exercising vigorously, your muscles may release more heat than your body is able to unload. The body temperature continues to rise and the rectal temperature, which is the same as the internal body temperature, may rise to over 104°F (40°C). The thermostat may reset to accommodate a higher temperature during prolonged vigorous exercise, just as it is believed to do when you have a fever. In any case, heat production and heat loss may increase to more than 20 times that noted at rest.

If the energy used with exercise exceeds the energy available in your diet, your brain stimulates you to eat more. In this way your brain helps you maintain a stable body weight. Of course, if you override the brain's stimulus to eat more through will power, you will lose weight. Exercise drives your calorie-balance system to eliminate calories. This stimulates your system to increase your calorie intake to keep up with the increased calorie requirements. Reducing your calorie intake shuts down your energy system, and decreases heat production.

If you use both together, in sensible manner, you can help your body maintain its proper weight. If you limit your calorie intake and also exercise vigorously, you can cause a negative calorie balance. By pushing yourself beyond what your body is designed for, you eventually force yourself into undernutrition, with its disastrous results. That is essentially what happened with the young men in the Minnesota experiment. They consumed 1,570 calories a day, but their physical activity and basic needs were much higher, so they were forced into undernutrition, with loss of fat-free body weight. As they lost metabolically-active tissue, they required fewer calories, but they experienced all the bad effects of undernutrition.

Muscles Make You Lean

The size of your muscles is important to you metabolically. About 40 percent of the body weight of an average adult is muscle. Even at rest, muscles still use 25 percent of the calories released by your body as heat. That is because muscles are metabolically-active tissue. It follows that the individual with more muscles will be able to eliminate more calories at rest than the individual with less muscle. That is why a 150-pound person, who is muscular and has very little fat, will use more calories than a 150-pound person with less muscle and more fat. Fat tissue (except brown fat) is almost inert in terms of using calories. Mostly, it is just a storage space for fat. That is why you do not want to shrink your metabolic tissue, such as your muscles. If you do, your near-basal calorie requirements will decrease. Then since you require fewer calories, you have to eat less to avoid having a positive calorie balance, and getting fat.

Of course, your muscles use far more calories once they start working. They can release heat simply by tensing. That is one of the first ways your muscles can help your body tolerate cold. As your body temperature starts to drop, you will automatically shiver, which simply escalates the amount of heat provided by your muscles.

Fueling Your Working Muscles

Inside your muscles are protein plates that literally slide over each other to cause muscular contraction. These are like sliding doors. As these plates slide over each other, your contracting muscle shortens, doing mechanical work, and releasing calories of heat. There are some high-energy compounds inside your muscles that provide the initial source of energy. That is very short-lived, and then your muscles must turn to other energy sources. The main source, after that initial burst of work, is the glycogen stored in your muscles.

Glycogen is really blocks of glucose that have been hooked together to form an "energy package" of glycogen. The glycogen is broken down to glucose, which is burned with oxygen to release carbon dioxide, water and energy. Your muscles need glycogen to be able to work. That is why it is so important to build up the glycogen stores in your muscles. If your glycogen stores are depleted, you will not have the energy to work your muscles. That is one reason why a person who is not accustomed to heavy muscular work will be able to work well one day, but will be tired the following day. It may take one or two days to replenish a muscle with glycogen before it can do as much work as before its glycogen stores were depleted. Most of the glycogen comes from the carbohydrates you have eaten. Some of it can come from conversion of some amino acids to glucose in the liver. That means your muscles can use some protein for fuel, as well as carbohydrate. As the glycogen stores in the working muscles are depleted, the liver glycogen is broken down and added to the blood glucose. The glucose in your blood is absorbed into your working muscles to replenish their energy supply. It is a little like putting another log on the fire.

As exercise continues beyond 10 minutes, the glucose and free fatty acids in your blood are absorbed and used by the working muscle. Since there is a relatively small amount of fat inside the muscle cells, it is not a significant source for the energy that must be provided. The fatty acids that are used for energy are mobilized from fat cells. These are transported by the circulation to the muscle cells for burning. As exercise progresses, more and more glucose and fatty acids are provided by the circulation to the working muscles to compensate for the diminishing muscle glycogen. The liver glycogen is broken down to glucose to maintain the blood glucose level. After four hours of work, about 61 percent of the energy for the working muscle comes from free fatty acids, transported to your muscles for burning. This tells you that prolonged exercise increases your body's use of fat, and consequently the mobilization of fat from fat deposits.

The amount of work your muscles can do is dependent upon the amount of oxygen provided by the circulation, and the available calorie supply in terms of glycogen, glucose and free fatty acids. Often, prolonged work will exceed the circulation's ability to provide enough oxygen to burn these hydrocarbons to carbon dioxide and water. Because this is a biological system, it has a wonderful mechanism that allows you to literally borrow oxygen. It is the lactic acid cycle. Your muscle cells are able to process glucose to lactic acid, to release some energy without using oxygen. This is the anaerobic phase of catabolism, meaning it proceeds without oxygen.

The catch is that your muscles cannot tolerate too much lactic acid. The excess lactic acid is picked up by the blood and removed. But eventually, as work continues, more and more lactic acid accumulates and causes severe fatigue. That limits the amount of work you can do. As you rest, and your circulation continues to pump blood at a furious pace, the oxygen supply catches up. The extra oxygen is then used to convert the lactic acid back to the original compound. This tricky maneuver is how one accumulates an "oxygen debt," and how it is repaid.

How Many Calories?

How many calories does exercise use? Everyone who plans on using exercise to help lose pounds of fat wants to know the answer. The question is posed by the lady who writes,

> DEAR DR. LAMB: I'm a 56-year-old woman and have gained about 25 pounds of ugly fat. I desperately want to lose this weight, but diets don't work for me. If I lose a little weight with a diet, I gain it right back. This time I want to do it slowly with exercise. My reasoning is that if a diet won't work, maybe I'm working on the wrong end of things and should try a program to eliminate calories rather than starving myself.
>
> I need to know everything there is to know about how exercise causes the body to lose calories. At least I would like some information on how many calories you lose with walking, running and riding a bicycle. Is there any way you can tell how many calories your body is using during exercise? How can I best start my exercise program? Are there other exercises I can do that will help me lose fat and keep it off?

There are many figures for the calorie cost of various activities, and many of them are wrong. Why? Because the energy cost of most activities has been measured only for a short time, and the real effects on your metabolic balance may last much longer. How long depends upon the intensity and duration of the exercise. As a bench mark you can use the figure for a 154-pound (70 kilogram) person. If he walked a mile, between the speeds of two and four miles and hour, he would use 60 calories more than he would use at rest. This figure is for walking on level ground with no adverse conditions. Often you will see a figure of 90 calories per mile quoted, but that includes the calories used at rest, in addition to the calories used in walking. If you used 90 calories an hour at rest, that would be 30 calories in 20 minutes. Walking one mile at a speed of three miles an hour would also require 20 minutes. It follows that the 60 calories for walking a mile plus the 30 calories used for resting equals 90 calories used while walking the mile in 20 minutes.

Many people think that speed makes a difference. It doesn't, unless you walk very slowly or very fast. Between the range of two and four miles an hour, it makes no difference. Most people walk within that range. You are dealing with quantities of energy and work. Work is force through distance, and that is why it is the distance, not the speed, that counts.

Some people are confused about speed and calorie requirements. They don't stop to realize that if you walked an hour at a speed of two miles an hour, the distance would be two miles, and if you walked an hour at a speed of four miles an hour, the distance would be four miles. In our example of 60 calories per mile, walking two miles would require 120 calories. But if you walked four miles, that would require 240 calories. In each instance that would be 60 calories a mile. You would use more calories an hour when you walked faster, but only because you were able to walk a greater distance in the same time frame. In terms of eliminating calories, it is better to emphasize distance rather than speed.

What about bicycling and energy requirements? Again, there are a lot of variables, but if you are outside, on the level, it takes about half as many calories a mile while bicycling as it does while walking. The invention of the wheel does have some efficiency benefits. If you jog or run at a reasonable speed, you will use about 1.5 times as many calories as if you were walking. You can then set up a nice relationship between calories used for the three different forms of exercise. You can assign a value of one for bicycling, two for walking and three for running or jogging. Or, stated another way, you will use twice as many calories walking as you will cycling, and three times as many calories jogging or running as you will cycling. Of course, if you run or cycle fast, these relationships are changed.

Are the calories used with a stationary bicycle the same as cycling outside? Many people would rather exercise inside and want to know if they can use it instead of walking, as this lady writes,

DEAR DR. LAMB: I am 58 years old and date a man 62. We frequently discuss exercise, but don't do much exercising. He maintains that walking is better than anything else. I agree from what I have read. However, since I do not live in an area where walking is safe, I say that riding a stationary bicycle with the pressure correctly adjusted is just as beneficial. He says it isn't. He also likes to golf in the summer and says that golfing gives him exercise as beneficial as walking a mile or two. I say it doesn't. Can you discuss these points?

That stationary bicycle question this lady asks cannot be answered with a simple yes or no, because there are too many variables involved. But you can adjust the resistance so that you use as many or more calories as you would walking. Some models will give you information on how much work is being performed. If you walk while golfing, you certainly can use as many calories as you would walking a mile or two.

Another way you can estimate how much work you are doing is to use your heart rate. It is closely related to how much blood your heart is pumping. If you know what your heart rate is while walking a mile at a speed of three miles an hour, you can compare this to your other activities. A more accurate way to know how many calories you are using is to measure the amount of oxygen your body consumes with work, but that might take hours and requires equipment you don't have to provide a real answer. You can see how your heart rate would work to answer this person's question.

DEAR DR. LAMB: Just what are the merits of a treadmill for walking exercises to regulate or increase my heartbeat as opposed to actually walking in the city streets for about one hour, three times a week? My doctor strongly suggested walking exercises to help lower my blood pressure as well as increase my well-being related to stress in one's life.

The first step this person should take is to measure his heart rate while walking a mile. The end of the walk is a good point. Then when he knows what that is, he can adjust his treadmill to walk fast enough to result in the same heart rate. Then he can continue to exercise at that level for the same length of time he would spend walking outside. The goal is to work enough to increase the work of the heart. The heart's work is increased because it has to deliver more blood to provide more oxygen to the working muscles. The muscles need the oxygen to act on the fuel to release calories for mechanical energy and in the process liberate about three times as much energy as heat, just like an engine gets hot when it is running. The heat is then eliminated through your skin.

There is a nice point about using a target heart rate too; as your level of physical fitness improves, you can do more and more work to achieve the same heart rate. That is true whether you are working on a treadmill, a rowing machine, a stationary bicycle or walking, jogging or running outdoors.

Incidentally, good studies show that exercise opens the small arteries and is very useful in lowering high blood pressure in some patients.

A popular exercise device that I'm often asked about is the "rebounder." Again you are faced with the concept that you need vigorous exercise to provide any help as opposed to the benefits you can obtain even from some exercise. The question is raised in this lady's letter.

DEAR DR. LAMB: Recently I purchased a rebounder. I really like working out on it. Sometimes I just run in place on it and other times I dance on it. I work out on it about 15 minutes twice a day. When I bought it I was told it would help me lose weight and improve my heart and lungs. Now some of my friends tell me that exercising on a rebounder is no good and it can't improve my fitness or help me lose weight. One of my friends who insists that rebounders are no good doesn't exercise herself and she needs to. I think she is just knocking it because she doesn't exercise herself. Could you comment on rebounders and whether they are any good or not?

The same point about using your heart rate applies. Any exercise that can raise your heart rate above its resting level is increasing your use of energy. The more the increase in heart rate and the longer it is elevated, the more calories you are using. But it is important to realize that you don't want to do so much more than you are used to doing that it can work your heart too much too soon.

Studies show that if you're in poor shape, as I expect this lady's friend is, then a rebounder is a good way to start to get in shape. The rebounder does absorb a lot of the shock by its springs and the springs do some of the work. Incidentally, that is not all bad. People who have arthritis and don't want to jar their joints may find it helpful. A rebounder, as commonly used, provides as much exercise, or perhaps more, depending on how you use it, as walking does. Neither a rebounder nor walking will train you to compete in the Olympics but both are helpful.

Often, people think that if you can only eliminate 60 calories for each mile, walking cannot be very efficient in eliminating unwanted pounds of fat, or preventing fat deposits. That would be true if you planned on doing it all in one week, but that is not the sensible way to lose weight or to exercise. You need to think of it as an everyday activity. If you walked one mile every day, that would be 21,900 calories eliminated in a year. While you do not convert fat to muscle, and you will use glycogen for the exercise, the calorie balance ends up the same. So you can equate the negative calorie balance of 21,900 to pounds of body fat. Since there are 3,500 calories in a pound of body fat, walking a mile each day uses the calories present in 6.25 pounds of body fat in a year. If you grow muscles at the same time, you may not see this on the bathroom scales, but that will be the calorie change, and the body fat you could lose. It follows that if you walked two miles a day, you would eliminate the calories in 12.5 pounds of body fat; three miles a day, 18.75 pounds and four miles a day, 25 pounds in a year. For most people, a year's program at this level will get rid of all the excess body fat they should eliminate on a do-it-yourself program. It's slow. It's sure. And it is much safer than a crash-diet or crash-exercise programs.

Calorie Loss After Exercise

One of the points made by many health clubs and exercise facilities is that the exercise will increase your loss of calories the rest of the day. This has caused some disagreements, as is evident in this woman's letter.

DEAR DR. LAMB: I want to lose some weight this year. I am convinced that exercise is a better way to lose weight than trying to starve yourself. I'm not going to tell you how much I weigh, but I do need to lose about 20 pounds.

I was told at a health club that you lose calories for hours after you have exercised. My husband says that is not true and that you only lose calories while you are exercising. I had hoped that a good exercise program each morning would be just what I need to perk up my metabolism all day. Is he right that I'm getting a bill of goods at the health club?

Even a small amount of physical activity will increase your heat production and oxygen use. That is why it is so important to keep a person absolutely quiet before measuring his basal metabolism. The excitement of riding from home to the clinic for the test can affect the results. That is why doctors have the subject rest quietly in a darkened room for some time before the test. In view of this observation, it is not surprising that even light activity during the day will cause you to eliminate calories. You do not need to exercise at very high levels to drive your calorie-balance system. This point is evident from a study done in 1960.

The experiment consisted of walking 10 miles at a speed of four miles an hour, on a treadmill, while in the fasting state. The metabolic rate of the subjects increased to five times its value at rest. It stayed an average of 15 percent above the basal level for the next six hours. This tells you also why you cannot measure the calorie effect of exercise by just measuring the energy used during the activity. The calorie elimination effect continued for at least six more hours. Unless you had a great need to eliminate calories in a short span of time, and were in shape for it, most people would not, and should not, walk continuously for 10 miles. But for the person who has a serious overweight problem, and can build up walking long distances, this can be a great aid in eliminating calories.

More vigorous exercise will have a longer effect on calorie elimination. In another study, a subject exercised for 80 minutes at 75 percent of his maximum capacity. That is a lot of exercise. At 12 hours after the exercise was over, his energy requirement was still 19.3 percent higher than at rest before exercise.

Paul Pacy and colleagues of the Nutrition Research Group, Clinical Research Centre, Harrow, United Kingdom, studied the energy effects of milder exercise. Two young, healthy men and two young, healthy women, who were not overweight, exercised for 20 minutes on a stationary bicycle at levels of 35 to 55 percent of their maximum capacity to utilize oxygen. That represented an energy requirement of 3.6 times that at rest. Even at 40 minutes after exercise, the oxygen consumption, and hence the calorie requirement, remained at 13 percent above the resting level. The subjects exercised again for 20 minutes, and at 40 minutes after the second exercise period, their energy requirements were 22 percent above the levels required before the first exercise period. This study emphasizes again that moderate physical activity can significantly increase your body's ability to eliminate calories for some time after the exercise has ceased.

Some scientists have reported that you do not have an increased use of calories after you finish exercise. But you have to read carefully to realize they are not talking about the point made here. It is quite true that with moderate levels of exercise there will be no increased use of calories the following morning. That is a long enough time interval to miss the increased metabolism that occurs with mild exercise. How long and how much your energy requirement is increased is strictly a function of how long and how vigorous your exercise is. At first, when a person has poor exercise tolerance, he cannot safely exercise at a very high level or for very long. But as his level of physical fitness improves, he can exercise longer at higher levels. As this occurs his energy requirements after exercise will be more and will last longer.

You can take a cue from these studies about the type of exercise you might do to stimulate your energy system to release calories. A short interval of exercise every hour should keep your system above the resting level throughout the day. I must warn you, though, that *if you are not accustomed to exercising, don't plunge into frequent, short periods of exercise. Instead, begin slowly and do perhaps one session the first day, then gradually build up the frequency of your exercise without tiring yourself.* You can see from these studies that you do not have to be a marathon runner to obtain benefits from exercise and stimulate your energy-balance system.

Exercise Saves Your Muscles

The anabolic effects of exercise are an important part of its effects on your calorie-balance scheme. Exercise not only enables you to increase the elimination of calories of heat from the work itself, but it can be used to stimulate the growth of metabolically-active muscle. It is that effect which enables you to use exercise to prevent loss of muscle when you are on a diet. It is inevitable that if you are inactive, and simply reduce your calorie intake to establish a negative calorie balance, you will lose body protein. That includes some of your muscle— even heart muscle. If you exercise adequately, you can prevent that.

A study by W. B. Zuti and L. A. Golding a few years ago showed this fundamental relationship. They studied 25 women between the ages of 25 and 42, who were from 20 to 40 pounds overweight. All of them were studied for 24 days before a program to induce negative calorie balance was started. They were weighed to the nearest ounce. Their skinfold measurements were done with a sophisticated method at the cheek, chest, mid-axillary, umbilicus, iliac crest (top of pelvic bone), rear thigh, interior thigh, lateral thigh and calf area, to estimate their percent of body fat. Also, they were carefully studied by water immersion. The total body fat was subtracted from the total body weight to establish how much of their body weight was not body fat—the lean body weight.

After these careful studies, the women were divided into three groups. The diet group had their calorie intake set at 500 calories less than they needed to maintain their body weight at their same level of activity. The exercise group stayed on the standard diet, but increased their exercise enough to equate to using 500 calories. The combination group decreased their dietary intake 250 calories and increased their exercise level enough to account for 250 calories of energy. In this way, all three groups had a negative calorie balance of 500 calories. The program was continued for 16 weeks. The diet-only group lost an average of 11.7 pounds (5.3 kilograms), the exercise group, 10.6 pounds (4.8 kilograms) and the combination group, 12.0 pounds (5.5 kilograms).

One of the most interesting aspects of this study was what happened to the lean body weight. The diet-only group lost 2.42 pounds (1.1 kilograms) of lean body weight. The combination group actually gained 1.0 pound (0.45 kilograms). But the exercise group gained 2.0 pounds (0.91 kilograms) of lean body mass. This study shows that the subjects who just dieted lost active metabolic tissue while exercise prevented it, even though it was fairly low-intensity exercise.

The point to learn from this study is that if you really need to lose pounds of fat, you should combine exercise with your diet program. It probably does make a difference what kind of exercise. It should include something of low intensity such as walking, but it should also include an overall exercise program that uses all of your muscles, to ensure that some muscles don't enlarge at the expense of muscles that are losing protein. This study shows that you can change body composition, not just lose pounds. The best result of a readjustment of your calorie-balance system is to increase your muscles while you are losing fat.

Exercise and Cold

Since exercise stimulates the heat-loss mechanism, it should be avoided if you are in a survival situation in the cold. That is why people are advised to stay in one spot and wait for rescue. If you exercise, you may feel warmer, because more hot blood will be circulating through your skin. But that rapid heat loss will exhaust your energy stores in a short time. That will limit the number of days you can survive in such a situation. Almost all occupations that require working while exposed to cold will require an increased calorie intake to maintain body weight. As you exercise, and the body temperature rises with blood flowing through the skin at a high rate, you can actually feel quite comfortable in the cold. One may ski on a sunny day on the cold mountainside and feel quite comfortable, even when stripped to the waist. Layered clothing makes it possible for a person to shed clothing as the body heat increases, and makes excess clothing for warmth unnecessary. All of this supports the idea that if you exercise in the cold, the cold can help you eliminate calories faster. That is great for weight loss, but a hazard if you need to survive arctic conditions. When the whole body is warm, your hands and feet are warm, even if they are exposed to the cold. The blood vessels open up in the feet and hands, despite the cold exposure, to help warm them. In fact, it is difficult to warm the hands and feet after cold exposure unless the entire body is warmed.

Exercise in cold water is particularly interesting because water is 25 times as conductive of heat away from the body as ambient air. That is why survival time after being immersed in cold water is so short. There is a lot of individual difference because this is one place where a layer of body fat helps. It provides a lot of insulation. It helps to keep the internal body heat from escaping. Exercise can maintain heat production in a relatively obese person in cold water. Studies of swimmers who have crossed the English channel estimate they expend 550 calories per hour in water at 4 degrees C (39 F). That is far more energy than the average person could be expected to expend over a prolonged period of time.

You can get another idea on the effects of cold water from the observation that a trim athlete will use 9 times the normal oxygen consumption when immersed in 10 degree C (50 degree F) water. A moderately obese person will maintain his internal temperature at normal levels with only twice the normal range of oxygen consumption. The insulation effect of fat can significantly improve a person's survival time if immersed in cold water, a point well substantiated by survival statistics in people who have been.

Starting Your Exercise Program

How can you start an exercise program to improve your calorie balance? I have tried to be very careful to show you that you do not need to perform high-intensity exercises to stimulate your calorie-loss mechanism. Of course, if you are an Olympic runner already, you won't need any help in this department, but if you are relatively inactive and overweight, you need to follow some general precautions. Almost everyone, except those who are sick in bed, can do some exercise. Those who can't walk already know it. For the vast majority, the best exercise is simply to start a walking program. If you can't walk outdoors, you can dance around in your living room at a slow pace for a short time. For the very inactive, a walk down the block and back may be it. After that, you can start doing it twice a day. Then you can gradually increase your distance and the frequency of your walks. If your are riding a stationary bicycle, peddle a few minutes at a comfortable speed without too much effort, then stop. Over the next days, weeks and months, you can gradually increase the amount. If you can just build up to three or four 20-minute exercise periods a day, that will do wonders toward stimulating your calorie-balance system. Never exert so much that your heart rate is rapid. If you want to condition your heart and lungs, you may want to exercise at more vigorous levels, but the goal we are discussing here is simply using exercise to help stimulate your calorie-balance system.

In terms of your energy-system it is probably better to do light exercise, such as walking at a comfortable speed, for a long period of time than it would be to run. If you could walk for four 20-minute periods a day at a speed of three miles an hour, that would be four miles a day. That will use about 240 extra calories. But if you ran a mile, that would use about 90 calories. There are a lot more people who can walk a mile four times a day than can run a mile. Never let anyone mislead you into thinking that walking isn't good for you. It depends on what you want to use it for. If you want the benefits of losing excess pounds of body fat, it is one of the best exercises that most people can do without being uncomfortable, or overexerting to the point that it could be harmful to them.

Some people believe you have to sweat to lose weight. That is not true. However, in comfortable weather, when you begin to sweat, it means that your exertion has reached the point that it has significantly turned on the heat-loss mechanism. That means you are losing more calories through your skin than if you were not warm or sweating.

Obviously, the higher the level of physical effort you can sustain, the more calories you will eliminate.

Don't Exhaust Your Brain

A word of caution is in order about the relationship between physical exertion and mental work. A short break devoted to exercise, away from office work or mental tasks, will stimulate a person and may improve his productivity. More exercise may not. It is that old problem in biology; just because a little is good doesn't mean that more is better. The right amount of exercise will make you feel better and energize you. But remember what happens as you continue to work your muscles and they use more and more glucose. As this continues, you can significantly diminish your glycogen stores. If you exhaust yourself with too much physical effort, you may compromise the glucose available for your brain. Or your body will be using a lot of your protein to form glucose. At that point, your brain may not function at its top level. Using it is like trying to run your computer without enough electrical energy. It doesn't work as well. *If you want to be able to make your best mental effort, the key is to exercise the right amount to stimulate your body, but not enough to exhaust it.*

Summary 12

1. Exercise turns on your metabolic furnace and liberates calories of heat. That is why people sweat if they exercise vigorously. Dieting shuts down your metabolic furnace and can make you feel cold, causing you to use fewer calories.
2. Lack of exercise can make you fat. Livestock managers use this concept by penning livestock to prevent exercise while fattening them.
3. About 75 percent of calories used to do exercise are liberated as heat through your skin. Only 25 percent is used as mechanical energy to do the work.
4. Too few calories combined with lots of exercise can cause undernutrition, just as starvation does.
5. Your muscles use energy even at rest and the more muscle you have the more calories you can use at rest.

6. A 154-pound person will use about 60 calories more when walking a mile than sitting still for the same time.

7. At most normal walking speeds the number of calories used is dependent on the distance walked, not the speed.

8. As a convenient rule, you use twice as many calories when you are walking as you do cycling and three times as many calories jogging or running slowly as you do cycling.

9. Your heart rate while exercising is a convenient way to evaluate how much energy you are using with a variety of exercises.

10. People do continue to use more calories after the exercise is over than they do at rest. How much and for how long depends on how vigorous the exercise is and how long it lasts.

11. Exercise, when limiting calorie intake, helps to prevent loss of lean body weight. That is one reason why exercise should be part of every calorie restricted diet program.

12. Exercise in the cold, particularly cold water, will speed up the loss of calories through the skin.

13. The right way to start an exercise program for those who are not accustomed to exercise is very slowly, usually with a walking program, then gradually increase the amount and frequency.

14. Light exercise stimulates you and enables you to do mental work better afterward. Exercise that exhausts you decreases your mental ability temporarily. It uses the glucose for exercise that you need as energy for your brain.

Chapter 13

Putting Your Muscle into Your Calorie Balance

DEAR DR. LAMB: I am a lady in my later 40s and for years I have battled my weight. I'd take off 15 pounds and put on 25. I'd try exercising, but having small children and always being in a hurry I didn't take the time to exercise on a regular basis.

I developed so much flab that I shook all over when I walked. My upper arms jiggled terribly. My stomach was loose and my legs were flabby.

About 10 months ago I bought some weights, about two-and-a-half pounds for my legs and wrists. I also got small dumbbells that ladies use. I started doing a few exercises with weights each exercise session. Now I can do a lot of exercises using my weights.

I'm not kidding myself. I have my share of wrinkles and look my age, but I'm so proud that I have firmed myself. It's such a nice feeling. I don't jiggle when I walk any more. The funny thing is, people think I have lost weight, but I haven't. I am 5 feet 4 and weigh 140 pounds and no one believes it.

A life of Lean Cuisine and salads is not for me. I like everthing. Exercise is the thing for me. It takes time, but if women would try it for two or three months, they could feel the difference. It's such a nice feeling not to pinch an inch or two at my waistline now. I hung over bad a few months ago.

One of the most neglected aspects of using exercise to adjust your calorie balance is developing and maintaining your muscles, as this lady has discovered. As I mentioned earlier, your muscle size has a lot to do with how many calories your body uses, even under near-basal conditions. It is plain folly to go on a low calorie diet because you weigh more than the tables say you should weigh, when that increased weight is caused by muscle development. You can help yourself stay lean, but not always lighter, by developing your muscles. You can cause yourself to be at risk of getting fat by allowing your muscles to deteriorate. It is important to have some level of endurance exercises in your lifestyle, such as walking, or jogging if you are in shape for it, but endurance exercises are not the answer to total body fitness, nor are they the only way you can exercise to help maintain a healthy calorie-balance system. Endurance exercises have their greatest effect in helping you eliminate calories by driving your catabolic system. Strength exercises help you through their anabolic action in building muscles, which, in turn, increases your near-basal calorie requirements.

Age and Muscle Size

One of the best examples of what can happen is available from the studies of the man who defined basal metabolism in 1906, Magnus Levy, a British physiologist. He measured his basal calorie requirements at age 26 and it was measured again at age 76. The results were as follows:

	Weight	cal/hr	cal/24-hr
Age 26	67.5 kg (148.5 pounds)	67	1,608
76	60.0 kg (132 pounds)	52	1,248
	7.5 kg (16.5 pounds)	15	360

At age 26, evidently he was not overweight, and he needed about 1,608 calories for his near-basal energy requirements. That is a fairly normal figure which one would expect for a young person in average physical condition. But notice that at age 76, some 50 years later, he was 16.5 pounds lighter and he used only 1,248 calories for his basal energy requirements.

It is safe to assume that he probably did not develop more muscles between the ages of 26 and 76. In fact, you can calculate his fat-free body weight. Remember the point that a kilogram of fat-free body weight required 1.28 calories an hour under near-basal conditions? You can divide that figure into the cal/hr figure and you will know his fat-free body weight in kilograms, which happens to be 52.34 kg, at age 26

(67 cal/1.28 = 52.34 kg (115 pounds),
and 40.62 kg, at age 76
(52 cal/1.28 = 40.62 kg (89.4 pounds).

Since you know what his total body weight was, you can calculate his percent of body fat, which was 22 percent at age 36 and 32 percent at age 76. Those, too, are not unexpected figures for those different ages, unless he had followed a strength training program in later years. It is true that without an exercise program which uses some form of strength exercises, your muscles will get smaller as you get older, from disuse and from loss of muscle units. Notice that Magnus Levy achieved energy equilibrium at both weights. When he was young, he weighed more and required more calories. When he was 76, he weighed less and required fewer calories. The body weight and energy requirements tend to reach equilibrium and then the weight remains stable, whether you are consuming lots of calories and weigh a lot or whether you are thin and use few calories.

What effect did the loss of fat-free body weight have on Magnus Levy's calorie requirements? It decreased his daily energy requirement 360 calories at age 76, compared to age 26. Unless he increased his daily level of activity, he would need to eat less or gain weight in the form of body fat. He would have to walk at least six miles a day just to use the same number of calories that he used for near-basal calorie requirements when he was 26 years old and not gain fat deposits. How do you know that? Walking a mile would not have used more than an additional 60 calories, and he needed 360 calories less for his near-basal calorie needs at age 76. So, 360 divided by 60 is 6 miles.

This is a very good illustration of the importance of muscle size. Had Magnus Levy been able to maintain the same fat-free body weight he had at age 26, he would not have needed to walk 6 miles a day when he was 76 to use the same number of calories. Strength exercises that maintained, or even increased, his muscle size throughout his life would have helped him avoid this decrease in calorie requirements. You can avoid this problem by including strength exercises in your program to maintain your muscle size as you go through life. These are not endurance exercises, such as walking, but exercises that cause your muscles to work against resistance.

When you walk, jog or run, your leg muscles do most of the work. They will get just large enough to support your body weight. The resistance they work against is your weight. If you look at champion runners, they tend to have lean well-muscled legs, while the rest of their muscular development usually is not at an equal level.

Building Muscle

What can you do to develop your muscle size? Weight lifting is the classical way. It goes back to the ancient story of the young man who grew strong by lifting a small bull calf each day. As the bull grew, so did the young man, until by the time the bull was full grown, the young man's body was bulging with muscles. It is a quaint story, but it embodies the basis for developing muscle size and strength. A muscle grows as it is forced to work against progressively increasing resistance. It will only grow as large as it needs to be to do a specific task. If your arm lifts nothing heavier than a martini, you are apt to have martini muscles. But if you lift weights, in increasing amounts, your arm muscles will increase in size as the weight increases.

Regardless of your program, you will not develop larger muscles unless your work them against resistance. It need not be a weight. It can be one of the machines that offers resistance as you work your muscles against it. Don't overlook using your own body weight as a means of developing and maintaining a reasonable amount of muscle size and strength. You accomplish a lot of that with a variety of calisthenics. Doing chin-ups will help develop the muscles in your shoulders, and so on. *A major reason people gain weight as they get older is because they lose muscle strength and size but continue to consume the same number of calories*. Their TV muscles are not large enough to require many calories. Since most people spend more time sitting than they do exercising their muscles, it becomes apparent that it is important to have a musculature that will use a lot of calories while you sit. The good thing about this is, that once you have developed a good set of muscles, it really doesn't require a lot of time to maintain them.

How do you develop a good set of muscles? There are factors that will limit your development that you do not control, such as inherited characteristics, but many people fail because they use the wrong approach, and are short on patience. There have been many studies to find out exactly what you have to do to get the best results in developing muscles. How much weight should you use? How often should you do the exercises? The best opinion seems to be that you should use a weight that your muscles can move through their range of motion by contracting at least three times, and not more than 10 times. Or, if you are using a machine, it should be set so that you can contract your muscles against resistance at least three times, but no more than 10 times. If you use a weight that you can lift five times, that is called a 5 RM load. When you lift the weight five times, that is called a set. If you do one set with a 5 RM load, rest and do another 5 RM set, that is the maximum you need to do with that muscle to stimulate it to develop.

As your muscle develops, you progress to doing 10 contractions with 5 RM weight. When you can do two sets at this level, it is time to increase the weight, so that your muscle has to work against an increased load again. By repeating and repeating this procedure over a period of time, always with progressively increased resistance, your muscle will be stimulated to develop. The more weight, or the greater the resistance, the bigger the muscle will be. Now, you don't have to develop a body like Arnold Schwarzenegger to benefit from strength training, any more than you have to be able to run a 26-mile marathon to benefit from endurance exercises. A good program with light weights can go a long way toward developing and maintaining your muscle size.

I receive a lot of letters, from young men in particular, telling me that despite their vigorous workout, they have not been able to develop larger muscles. Young men often want to "muscle-up," and not being able to is a distinct disappointment to them. This is a typical letter from a parent.

> DEAR DR. LAMB: Our son is 15 years old. He is trying to gain weight. He is 6 feet tall and weighs 140 pounds. He plays basketball every day, does weight lifting and runs a mile every day. He eats like a horse and drinks milk shakes for extra calories, yet has a difficult time gaining. Any suggestions would be appreciated.

Often, the problem is from being too strongly motivated. This young man is probably overdoing his exercise program. Growing muscles has some things in common with growing plants. It takes time. If a person greatly exceeds the two-set level for strength exercises, his muscles will not grow. All you want to do is stimulate the muscle adequately, then let it rest, so it has time to respond to that stimulus. Many people active in bodybuilding like to say that you "tear down" the muscle one day and let it "build up" the following day. That is not quite accurate, because the exercise need not tear down the muscle, but it does take a day in between exercises to allow your muscle to grow. If you work it again the following day, you deprive it of growing time. Also, if you work your muscle for 5, 10 or more sets, those additional sets simply exhaust the muscle so that its growth is slowed. All that activity this young man is doing, plus the calories used for growth, means there is a limit to what's left for muscle development. Also at age 15 he may not yet have had all the effect on his muscles that will occur from the testosterone levels he will produce in the next few years. Testosterone does stimulate the development of muscles and that increases the amount of metabolically active tissue a male has.

Another point is important to remember. *It is now popular to say, "no pain, no gain." That is completely wrong. If you have pain, you are not likely to gain.* Muscle pain with an exercise program, whether from endurance exercises or strength exercises, means that you have done too much. That muscle soreness is because of injured muscle. Electron microscopic studies shows the injury and necrosis (death) of muscle tissue in that state. You want to use an exercise program that stimulates muscle growth, not one that causes necrosis of muscle tissue.

Age No Barrier

It is sometimes said that you can't increase your muscle size and strength as you get older. That is not true. But if you have blocked arteries that cannot increase the blood flow to a muscle, then you can't exercise the muscle enough to get the best results. Also, if you damage the nerve fibers to a muscle, it may atrophy. You can see this in the leg muscles of a person who has had a ruptured intervertebral disk that has been allowed to press on spinal nerves too long.

Otherwise, developing an old muscle is just like developing a young muscle. The muscle fibers will enlarge as they are worked against resistance. A physical education specialist, John P. O'Shea, proved how this worked for him. He was 50 years old and had been a former competitive weight lifter, but he had not done any lifting for 16 years. He began a strength-training program. After a year, there was an improvement in his squat of 80 percent; his dead lift, 66 percent and his bench press, 48 percent. His body also showed the increased muscular development. Don't let anyone discourage you about the value of strength training as you get older. You may need to be more careful and progress slower, but you can do it.

Diet Is Important

It takes more than just stimulation with exercise to develop good muscles. You do need good nutrition. I am often asked if various protein powders will help to stimulate muscle development. Consider the young man who wrote,

> DEAR DR. LAMB: I am 20 years old, 6 feet 4 inches tall and weight 170 pounds. I want to build muscle in hopes of becoming a professional wrestler and would like your advice on how I should start a weight lifting program. How often and how long should I lift each time? I know you can overwork your muscles.
>
> I have been told to use a weight gain growth and training mix, which has many different vitamins along with protein and carbohydrates.

This young man does not need a lot of expensive protein powders, or any other commercial product. For muscle development you need a good diet to provide sufficient calories and good quality protein. For every pound of lean muscle you develop, your body will need to store an additional 100 grams of protein. That figure is based on the fact a pound of lean beef muscle contains 100 grams of protein. If you grew a pound of lean muscle a week, your body would need to retain an additional 100 grams of protein a week, or about 15 grams a day. Let's consider the point that your body is not a perfect chemical machine and will not efficiently convert 15 grams of extra protein in your diet directly into lean muscle. As a safety factor, you can triple that 15-gram figure. In that case, you would want 45 additional grams of protein a day. For an active, growing young man the maximum protein he will need according to the RDA values is 56 grams a day. If you add the two figures (45 and 56) you will find that 101 grams of good quality complete protein a day in your regular diet should adequately support the development of a pound of lean muscle a week.

How can you get 100 grams of good quality protein a day? That is rather easy. A quart of protein-fortified skim milk, which you can find in most grocery stores, will contain about 40 grams of good quality protein. If you used regular milk, it would contain a little less. For the other 61 grams you can use about two-thirds of a pound (flesh only) of lean items from the meat group, which could include breast of chicken, lean round steak, fish or other items from the group. Most people will not have any trouble eating that small quantity of food from the meat group each day. I have included the protein content with the items in the meat group and dairy group of the basic diet I suggested you could use to develop your diet plan.

There is another dietary requirement to help you build muscles. *You need enough calories.* If you do not have enough calories in your diet to meet your calorie needs, some of that protein in your diet will be used for calories rather than to build more muscle. That is another reason why many of the young men I hear from can't develop muscles. In addition to their muscle-building program, they are often active in many other sports. If they run several miles a day, and are active in other ways, all that activity will also require calories. When the calorie use exceeds the level of calorie consumption, there will not be any significant muscle growth. If you are overweight, and have stored calories of fat, these can be used for part of your calorie requirements while you are building muscles. That is how a person's body composition is changed to less fat and more muscle.

There are a number of recommendations for diets for muscle development that are really bad for you. You need the elements in your diet I have discussed, but you don't need expensive protein supplements or other gimmicks. It is a mistake to consume a lot of fat. You can get your calories from carbohydrate. Fat is not used in growing muscles. Excess fat consumption, as can occur from the practice of drinking half-and-half cream, may significantly increase your fatty-cholesterol particles and contribute to heart disease, or even strokes. Heart attacks can occur at an early age. You do not need a lot more calories than required for your energy needs and muscle-building program. If you consume lots of extra calories, you will have fat deposits like anyone else. For those interested in developing a nice-looking body, surrounding your new muscles with a layer of fat is not the way to go.

Another terrible dietary habit, sometimes practiced, is to eat a lot of eggs. Since an egg yolk contains from 220 to 250 mg of cholesterol, that means a very high-cholesterol diet. Heart specialists recommend limiting your cholesterol from all sources to no more than 300 mg a day. That includes the cholesterol in meat and milk that you need. If you follow the dietary suggestions I have made, you can achieve this. A high-cholesterol, high-fat diet can result in a sick, diseased heart muscle, regardless of how good your skeletal muscles may look.

An important final point needs to be made about nutrition and muscle development. While nutrition is essential to good muscle development, nutrition alone will not cause a person to develop a good set of strong muscles. That requires the right genes and the right exercise program to stimulate its development. Exercise is the main stimulus to development.

Hormones and Amino Acids

There are some other bad practices used to develop muscles. The one the public is most aware of is the use of steroids. Can you help build muscle by using steroids? Yes. There is some disagreement about how effective they are, but the anabolic steroids are chemically developed hormones similar to testosterone which do not have all of testosterone's sexual effects. That doesn't mean they have no effect in this department. The use of these early in life may limit growth in height. There are many dangerous side effects, including liver disease, sterility from lack of formation of sperm cells and others, but the one that I find most disturbing is not often mentioned. Testosterone is the factor that suddenly increases the total cholesterol levels in males when they reach puberty and testosterone is the reason they produce a lot more LDL-cholesterol that leads to heart attacks. The use of steroids may increase these factors, and while a man is developing better muscles he may be progressing to a heart attack. I have had letters from friends of young men who have had fatal heart attacks after such a program. Add to this the dietary problems I just mentioned of consuming lots of saturated fat and cholesterol and you have a time bomb ticking away while skeletal muscles are growing.

Some women athletes have also used steroids. Remember that one reason men tend to have more muscular bodies than women is because men produce more testosterone. It is not surprising that when women use steroids they may develop masculine characteristics, including such things as increased hair development in the wrong places.

Then there is a new danger on the horizon and that is the use of growth hormone. Remember that growth hormone comes from the pituitary. For years that was not a significant problem because it could only be obtained from human pituitary glands and they were in very short supply. There was a limited amount that could be used to treat children with insufficient growth because of growth hormone deficiencies. But in recent years it has become possible to synthesize growth hormone and the supply is no longer limited. Already there is a black market for this hormone to help people who want to be bigger. Growth hormone does help stimulate muscle growth. But without other active factors the muscles are weak.

There are several reasons why safe levels of growth hormone will never be the answer to growing larger strong muscles. When a person who produces a normal amount of growth hormone takes additional growth hormone, the body's natural output is decreased enough to make up for the medicine a person takes. If you take even larger amounts you can cause serious side effects. Doctors have long been familiar with these changes, called acromegaly. The jaw and skull bones grow, causing an unpleasant change in appearance. The hands may double in size and have a spade-like appearance. The feet also become quite large. Diabetes often occurs. The nose may become enlarged to twice its previous size. None of these changes are the sort of thing that a person who wants to improve his body would really like to have.

There is some danger that young children may take growth hormone to increase their height. Parents are sometimes anxious to have a promising child become a basketball super star. While you can never be sure what a person's motivation is from a letter, you wonder when you get a letter like this one.

DEAR DR. LAMB: Our 13-year-old son wants to know what he can do to insure growth to the maximum height and size possible for his genetic makeup. He is very healthy and above average for his age at 5 feet 10 and 140 pounds. He eats everything in sight and gets plenty of rest and moderate exercise. He also takes vitamins. Is there anything else he can do to aid his growth? He wants to become a basketball or football pro and shows tremendous promise.

Notice that this letter comes from the father and not the boy. While bone age is the real criteria for determining future growth potential, at age 13 it is likely that this boy has a lot of opportunity to grow naturally without imposing the dangers of taking growth hormone.

A related problem is the use of amino acids. When you eat good quality proteins, you get a mixture of amino acids that your body is well designed to process. But taking large amounts of individual amino acids may have a quite different effect. The work in this area is definitely still experimental. You see ads to the effect that taking certain amino acids will help you "burn off fat while you sleep." The two amino acids often hawked for this purpose are arginine and ornithine. It is claimed that they will cause a release of growth hormone that will cause you to lose fat deposits and develop muscle. There is limited information available, but studies that are available on arginine taken by mouth suggest that a 150-pound person would have to consume 17.5 grams to have any effect on increasing the output of growth hormone, several thousand times the milligram quantities available in the usually marketed products. Considering the effects of the excess output of growth hormone, that is probably fortunate. Perhaps the only outcome of the use of these substances will be a waste of money.

How to Maintain Your Muscles

With a sensible strength-training program, and a sensible diet, most people can improve their muscle size and their health. Don't expect miracles overnight, but if you are patient over a period of months, you will succeed.

Once you have developed the muscles you want, how can you keep them? You shouldn't need extra protein anymore, unless you are going to develop more muscles. But you do need to keep stimulating the muscles at the maximum level of their capability. You can do that just one day a week to maintain the level of muscle development that you have achieved. If you don't exercise your muscles adequately once a week, they will decrease in size to just meet the requirements you ask of them. If that is just lifting a martini, you will soon be back to martini muscles again.

Summary 13

1. Increasing the size of your muscles through strength training helps prevent body fat accumulation. Muscles use calories even when they are not working.
2. As your muscles decrease in size, you use fewer calories.
3. The basis for increasing muscle size is to contract the muscles against resistance. The resistance is progressively increased as the muscle size increases.
4. Too much exercise, such as lots of running and sports, at the same time a person is trying to develop muscle size may prevent muscle development.
5. Muscle pain and soreness means muscle damage and decreases the results of an exercise program. No pain, no gain is wrong when it comes to muscle development.
6. Age is usually not a barrier to improving muscle size and strength.
7. A proper diet that provides sufficient complete protein is essential for your muscles to respond to strength exercises. Usually 100 grams of complete protein is adequate and that is easily supplied by the diet. That makes it unnecessary to buy expensive protein powders and supplements hawked to people wanting to build muscles.
8. The total calorie intake is important. You need enough calories to meet your energy needs so the extra protein will be available to build muscles.
9. There is no reason to consume foods that are bad for your health, such as lots of cream or eggs or other fatty foods. These can increase a person's risk of coronary heart disease.
10. Testosterone stimulates muscular development. Anabolic steroids have many of the actions of testosterone and will stimulate some muscle development at considerable risk to the individual, including increasing the risk of heart attacks in males. They cause women to become more masculine.
11. Growth hormone is sold on the black market. Extra growth hor-

mone either does not help a mature person develop muscles, or when available to the body in excess amounts causes severe and undesirable changes in the body, as does acromegaly in patients with diseases that produce excess growth hormone. Most of the growth hormone products sold on the black market are ineffective and some products are frauds.

12. Amino acids, arginine and ornithine, are marketed to promote muscle development and burn off fat. This is another scam, as the small amount in the products sold is far below the amount needed to stimulate the production of growth hormone by the body. Which may be fortunate.

Chapter 14

The Many Faces of Overweight

The identification of being thin with youth and beauty is of recent origin. Venus de Milo was a full-bodied woman. Cleopatra would not have placed in a fashion model contest today, and most of those Titian nudes of beautiful women of the times would be sent to the fat farm. Diamond Lil, who was considered a charmer in her day, and won five husbands, weighed 225 pounds. Beauty is clearly in the eye of the beholder, and today the beholder wants to see a slim silhouette.

Health has played an important role in our view of what is overweight. There is no doubt that being overweight from consuming too many calories and not getting enough physical activity has been a major factor in causing the epidemic of heart attacks and strokes in industrialized nations. Men began to weigh as much in their late twenties as previous generations weighed when they were in their mid-forties. The middle-aged spread began a little too early. Before the heart disease epidemic, it was considered unhealthy to be thin or lose weight. That is understandable, since in 1900 tuberculosis was the leading cause of death. Although fatty-cholesterol blockage (atherosclerosis or hardening of the arteries) was rarely observed at autopsies, heart attacks were so uncommon that the first case in a living person was not diagnosed until 1908. Since tuberculosis and cancer were the scourge of the land, most people learned to think of weight loss as a sign of poor health.

It wasn't until after World War II that the heart attack epidemic made people realize that being "pleasingly plump" might not be healthy. Slowly, as this fact was realized, and with tuberculosis under control, it became important to be thin. It is important to eliminate pounds of body fat if you have specific medical problems that predispose to heart attacks and strokes, such as high cholesterol levels, high blood glucose levels or high blood pressure. But the end result of the emphasis on being thin, particularly in a fashion-conscious society, is that millions of people in a state of negative calorie balance are suffering from undernutrition. Most of them do not know where their youthful vigor has gone. The simple truth is, "feeling good" has been replaced with "looking good." In many cases, it is really true that beauty is only skin deep. What is happening inside is unhealthy when you have starved your body. Many people are "looking good" on the outside, but not "doing good" on the inside.

There seem to be two extremes to the problem, being overweight and being underweight. Neither is particularly desirable. Not all people who seem to be overweight need to lose weight. One of the current difficulties in approaching the question of being overweight is the tendency to think that all people who are overweight get that way for the same reason. There are many reasons for being overweight, in the sense of having increased amounts of body fat, not just weighing more because you are well muscled.

I have spent a medical career learning new things about being overweight. In medical school I learned that obesity was always the result of eating too much. Remembering that gluttony is one of the seven deadly sins, it is easy to see why people who weighed more than our society thought they should weigh were often discriminated against. As I had to become more interested in problems of body weight because of its relation to medical problems I became fascinated with the differences I observed. I was fortunate enough to participate in the early days of seeking ways to prevent heart disease. When I became responsible for the medical examinations used in selecting the nation's astronauts, I was again concerned with the important factors of preventing heart disease.

There was, within the medical profession, a gradual awareness that there was more to losing weight than not carrying around candy bars in your purse or pigging out on eggs, bacon, mashed potatoes and gravy and fried foods. As the early diet studies began to evaluate the effects of high cholesterol levels, some wondered if the whole problem was not just that of too many calories of everything.

As society became even more conscious of weight problems, there was an unending parade of gimmicks to make you lose weight and books that proposed ridiculous ways for you to lose weight, including such temporary successes as *The Drinking Man's Diet*. But while evaluating the flight crews for the U.S. Air Force, I became impressed that the men having heart problems were the ones who were not only overweight but were also in a poor state of physical fitness. Their exercise capacity was well below what it should have been. Today I recognize that there are many different causes for being overweight. There is not just one problem that fits all. It is true that in some cases it is simply an excess intake of calories and not enough activity. This is often related to a lack of motivation, as this man's letter suggests.

DEAR DR. LAMB: I'm 31 years old, 6 feet 2 inches tall and weigh 225 pounds. My problem is weight gain and my seeming lack of motivation to do anything about it.

When I was in high school I was fat. When I graduated I went straight into the Marine Corps. Now those people have one helluva weight loss plan. Lose it or else. I shed weight like a hillside sheds water in a rainstorm. I went to boot camp weighing 235 pounds and came out three months later weighing 190. I looked and felt great. My self-esteem took a tremendous leap also. During my four-year tour in the Marines I maintained my weight at 190, which was not hard to do in such a structured environment.

Since then I have married, have one son and have settled into a very wonderful and happy life. But I regained weight and more recently I have been gaining at an alarming rate. I tell myself I have to get started eating better and get back to an exercise and weight training program. but I can't seem to get going anymore. I drive home envisioning myself exercising and doing all the things necessary to lose weight but when I get there I just want to sit and rest. How can I get motivated?

Sometimes it takes a shock to really motivate people to take the steps necessary to control their body fat. That shock may be a heart attack. Unfortunately, many people do not survive that first shock and really don't have a second chance. That is why it is so important to start. This man's description of his Marine life as "structured" is one key. Another is the motivation of others; that could include his wife, or it could include some of his men friends who want to improve their health as well. Motivation is what many organized efforts provide.

But where does he fit in the various causes of obesity. You can't know without a careful evaluation. Is he having a mild depression that saps his motivation? Does he need psychological help or even medication? Has he inherited a tendency to be fat? He could have more than one factor influencing his weight gain. These are the questions that have led me to formulate some beginning classification of the various causes for being "overweight."

The Overeaters

If you have extra fat you will probably be told it is because you are consuming too many calories. That is the simplest form of being overweight. In our society, with its abundance of calorie-rich foods, that is easy to do. Despite being born with a blueprint for average weight, an individual may override his calorie balance system by simply consuming too many calories. You can get a very good idea whether or not this is your problem by simply keeping a food diary. If you do not have access to information to help you calculate how many calories you are consuming a day, get some help from someone who can do this for you, like a dietitian. Just be certain that whoever you are working with doesn't have any misconceptions about how many calories you really need each day. You do need more than 1,200 calories a day. Look again at the daily calorie requirements that were discussed earlier. Remember that the recommended intake is 2,700 calories a day for a lean man who weighs 70 kilograms (154 pounds) and 2,100 calories for a woman who weighs 58 kilograms (128 pounds). That does not mean fat-free body weight or lean body weight, but the weight of a healthy person with a normal amount of body fat.

Finding out how many calories you are consuming may be very instructive. In the process, you may learn enough about the calorie content of foods, and how food preparation affects the number of calories, to help you adjust your eating habits. The choice of foods is often the problem, just as eating calorie-rich foods was the reason ordinary laboratory rats got fat.

There are some interesting characteristics of the person who is overweight because of overeating. This is a generalization and does not apply to the grossly obese, but it does apply to many who are moderately overweight. Since they are consuming more calories than they require, the excess calories cause the brain to turn on the metabolic furnace. That means the thyroid gland is working at its top level. Every mechanism the body has to process those calories is working. It is like turning your furnace up to its highest level and keeping it there. Of course, whatever the body cannot convert to heat and eliminate is stored as body fat. In animals, the brown fat is working hard to produce more heat and get rid of those calories. In humans, this may also be a factor. Remember that brown fat activity is stimulated by two things, cold and overeating.

With all those calories of heat being released, you might expect the body temperature to rise. But the brain's thermostat perceives the rising temperature, and turns on the heat-loss mechanism. It is a lot like what you would do if you were in a room that was getting too hot — turn on the air conditioner. The brain signals an increase in blood flow through the skin, to facilitate an increased loss of hot calories through radiation and convection. The sweat glands are stimulated to increase their action to speed up evaporation. That hot blood stimulates the temperature receptors in the skin, and the person becomes hot. Overeaters tend to be overweight and hot. They have a poor tolerance to hot weather because they are already working their system to unload heat. They sweat easily, and even a little physical exertion results in sweat rolling off their bodies.

Another characteristic of the overweight overeaters is their energy level. These people have an adequate supply of calories to drive their energy system. They may surprise you by not getting tired. Their muscles are full of glycogen for immediate work. Their liver is full of glycogen that can be mobilized for energy. They are travelling on a full tank of gas. You could say they are running their engine at full throttle.

Of course, the brain plays an important role in all of this. There are many reasons why a person wants to eat. The stimulated appetite ensures a steady input of excess calories for the metabolic furnace. Overeating, in terms of quantity, may be caused by psychological factors. It is no secret that when many people quit smoking, they have an increased urge to eat. How much of the overeating is from boredom, loneliness, for oral gratification, or some other factor, is not always clear. Certainly, altering a person's need to eat large quantities of food may help to stop overeating. That is where behavioral modification helps.

The overeaters are one of the group that often have significant medical problems. Frequently, they have driven their liver to produce an excess amount of fat (triglycerides) and cholesterol. Too much of this is packaged in the larger fatty-cholesterol particles, the low-density lipoproteins (LDL). The cholesterol in these particles is often called LDL-cholesterol. It is the kind that tends to lodge in the arteries and causes blockage of arteries to the heart, brain and other organs. It is a major factor in causing heart attacks and strokes. The other thing that happens to these overweight overeaters is high blood pressure. This, too, is a major factor in causing heart attacks and strokes. Clearly, those overweight overeaters who have high cholesterol levels and high blood pressure have ample reason to follow a program to reduce these important risk factors. That means a program that induces a negative calorie balance to correct their overweight condition.

The most obvious way to correct being overweight from overeating is to decrease the number of calories consumed. It is like turning down the furnace when the room is too hot. This should be done with a sensible, balanced diet that can provide the basis for a continued healthy eating pattern for life. Often, this means learning more about nutrition and foods, so that better choices can be made. It does not mean these individuals need to be on a starvation diet. In terms of eliminating excess pounds of body fat, it does not make any difference whether the decrease in calories is from decreasing the intake of carbohydrates, fat or protein. In terms of health, it is wise to cut out the fats. But you must decrease the total calorie consumption. There is no magic combination of foods that will enable you to beat the laws of nature. You may fool yourself by following some fad diet combination, but all diets ultimately cause you to lose body fat for only one reason—they decrease your calorie consumption. They provide fewer calories than your body needs. Don't be misled by the charlatans or the uninformed who would have you believe otherwise.

You can use the diet guide provided in chapter 11 to construct a diet that is suitable for you. Remember, that basic diet provides about 1,300 calories. It establishes the point that you can have a well-balanced diet that meets all your nutritional needs and consume only 1,300 calories a day. Such a diet will not provide all the calories you should have. But it can be helpful for the person who wants to lose a few pounds. Any diet that lasts more than a few weeks should provide more calories than that, or you risk developing undernutrition. You can use the basic diet plan to ensure that you will have a balanced diet, then add to it other food items of your choice. Do get a set of kitchen scales so you can weigh your portions, and know exactly what you are getting. That, too, can be an educational experience.

Do not go on a diet that promises quick weight loss. Those initial pounds of rapid weight loss are not from loss of fat, but from loss of salt and water. If you fall into that trap, you are just fooling yourself and abusing your body.

Keep in mind that decreasing your calories can cause you to lose body protein, such as muscle protein. Ultimately, that works against your success in avoiding excess body fat. You need to at least maintain your metabolically-active tissue, and it would be even better if you could stimulate it to an increase. You do that with exercise. If you have only a small amount of excess body fat, you may find that by controlling your calorie intake and increasing your exercise, in time, you can lose your pounds of excess body fat. Your brain will help you adjust your weight to its proper level. Every diet program should be accompanied with at least a light exercise program, such as walking, and, hopefully, with a set of general calisthenics that stimulate all the body's muscles.

Another important point—do not try to lose excess body fat too fast. It didn't get there overnight and you can't eliminate it safely overnight, either. You can avoid breaking down body protein by losing weight slowly. In most instances, a half-pound to a pound a week is fast enough. At that rate, your body will eliminate from 20 to 25 pounds in a year's time. That is adequate for most people. Those who need to lose more rapidly need medical supervision. I'm sorry to say that medical supervision will not guarantee that you will lose weight safely without abusing your body. The total concept of obesity and how to treat it is imperfectly understood, and often incorrectly applied. There are many doctors and nutritionists who are very capable of helping you with such a problem, but a large number of them depend solely on cutting your calories to the point that it is not good for your health.

The concept of undernutrition is not widely appreciated. Unfortunately, it doesn't cause a rash or a fever, and it cannot be detected with a cardiac catheter or a blood test. The most common early symptoms of undernutrition are fatigue, loss of energy and interest. Unfortunately, a well-motivated person who wants to lose weight may deny such symptoms. The professionals who are directing weight control programs often fail to ask about these symptoms, or may ignore them.

A bad diet that has been prescribed for you is no better than a bad diet you might construct for yourself. That is why you need to be knowledgeable about the basis of weight control. It is your self-protection against the widespread misinformation and lack of information on the subject.

Underactive Overweight

Our high-tech industrialized world, with its spectator sports and TV, has made it unnecessary to be physically active. Quite frequently, a person uses far fewer calories while at work than he does away from work. A wide variety of occupations involve sitting with little movement. It isn't just the typist who sits anymore. A high percentage of "factory" workers sit, as well. Others stand in one spot near a conveyer belt and are not required to do very much physical effort. Or executives spend their lives on the phone or in meetings. People don't chop wood anymore. If they cut wood, it is with a chain saw. Most of them don't even carry wood into the house. They just turn up the thermostat, or adjust their electric blanket. It is little wonder that we have a large number of people who do not use many calories from engaging in physical activity. The fitness boom has helped to offset this dismal fact, but it hasn't reached the many millions who are not motivated to be active.

Look again at what exercise does to your calorie balance system. It stimulates your energy system to release calories. It turns up your metabolic furnace. It stimulates the anabolic process for growth. It does a lot of other beneficial things as well, but, in terms of your calorie balance, these are its major effects. It is not surprising that without that stimulus, the body's muscles get smaller. The metabolically-active fat-free body gets smaller from disuse. Since your metabolic system is not being stimulated by exercise to release calories of heat, your heat-loss mechanism is not as active. The end result is that you consume more calories than your body uses. That causes a positive calorie balance and the excess calories are stored as body fat. That occurs even without consuming an excess of calories. The defect here is a failure to eliminate calories, rather than consuming too many.

Just as a daily log of your food intake is useful, so that you can estimate the number of calories consumed, it is equally important to keep a log of your activities. Such a log will give you some idea of the number of calories you are using a day. The two records together provide valuable information concerning the causes of being overweight—whether from consuming too many calories, inactivity or both.

The underactive overweight individual has several significant characteristics. He usually is not energetic. He is not functioning at full throttle like the overeating overweight individual. He may feel tired. One of the persistent observations from studies on inactivity is the fatigue it causes. A classic example is the person who stays in bed for a few days. Even if he is not sick, he will feel tired when he first gets out of bed and resumes activity. There is a whole gamut of symptoms and findings associated with inactivity. An office worker who sits all day comes home fatigued, but he or she often feels better after some light exercise. That activity stimulates the metabolic system and wakes it up, eliminating that sluggish feeling. The response to light exercise helps to separate this problem from undernutrition, camouflaged by genetic overweight. The overweight individual's history is of major importance in separating the two forms of fatigue. One has a history of an inadequate food intake, while the other has an adequate food intake, but a history of inadequate activity.

Some underactive overweight individuals may complain of feeling cold. That is not surprising, because their level of activity is so low that they are not stimulating heat production or heat loss. As a result, the blood flow through the skin is not increased and they do not feel hot.

These people do not need a new diet as much as they need an exercise program. Of course, they should follow a sensible balanced diet, but rather than try to eliminate pounds of body fat by severe calorie reduction, they need to slowly begin to increase their level of activity. A slow approach is particularly important in these people, because of the low levels of activity their body has adjusted to. A daily walking program is a good place to start. After that is underway, adding a very light calisthenic program is important. These people need to rebuild their endurance and their strength. They need endurance exercises to help burn off some of those calories stored as fat. They need calisthenics to help regain normal muscle size.

It is particularly bad to put these people on a severe calorie-restricted diet without exercise. That just increases the loss of their active metabolic tissue, including muscle, which simply exaggerates the problems already caused by inactivity. The best way to correct being overweight is to correct the problem that is causing it.

Underactive overweight people are also prone to have high cholesterol levels, low HDL-cholesterol levels (the good cholesterol) and elevated blood pressure. In this sense, they are not greatly different from the overeating overweight individual.

What if a person is both underactive and overeats? That combination is not exactly rare. He or she needs both a balanced, calorie-limited diet and a sensible exercise program.

Our underactive society has created a situation not unlike putting cattle in a feed-lot to fatten them. As mentioned earlier, limiting an animal's level of activity is an important part of fattening it. Humans are no different, and we need to avoid the feed-lot environment.

Genetic Overweight

For years, there has been an abundance of evidence that people inherit their tendency to be overweight or skinny. The animal kingdom demonstrates that with different breeds of cattle, horses and other animals. On a worldwide basis, you can see it in people of different ethnic origins. Some are small and thin, even with an adequate food intake. Others, such as the Hottentots, are genetically predisposed to having large fat deposits over the buttocks. The role of genes in determining our characteristics is evident everywhere. Being overweight tends to occur in families. It goes further than that. Even where the fat is deposited is a family characteristic—shades of the Hottentots. For several generations in some families, the women tend to have exceptionally large amounts of fat deposited over the thighs, and few, if any, fat deposits above the waist. The simple truth is there is a a reason why daughter looks like mother, and the reason is genetic. For the same reason, the old saying, "like father, like son" applies to more than just behavior.

The recently reported study of body weight in people who had been adopted, compared to the body weight of their genetic parents and their adopted parents, which I discussed earlier, is strong evidence for the important role of inherited genes in determining whether a person will be fat or lean. It is important to recognize this, as it makes a difference in how people function and how they should manage their diets and lifestyles.

Put simply, your brain has a predetermined level for how fat your body should be. You can override this range by what you do with your eating and exercise habits, but only with some difficulty. If you are thinner than you are supposed to be, all the brain has to do is turn down your metabolic furnace, and allow more calories to be stored as body fat. At the same time, it will shut down your heat-loss mechanism to maintain your body temperature. All the body's weight-control mechanisms it uses to defend its proper weight can be brought into play to keep you within your proper—or genetically predetermined—range.

How can you recognize that you have genetic obesity? That is still difficult, but your family history is a good start. If both of your parents were obese, you have an 80 percent chance of having genetic obesity. If both of your parents were lean, it is less likely. Look at your grandparents as well.

Many people who appear to be overweight actually feel fine. They may not have elevated blood pressure readings, high cholesterol levels or high blood glucose levels. If they do, these will need to be treated, and part of that treatment may require making a major effort to eliminate body fat. When people who have genetic obesity begin a program to lose weight, it is very difficult for them to do so. They are fighting their body.

Despite being overweight, they may have a normal level of physical activity and a perfectly normal calorie consumption. They may not have any sensations of being either too hot or too cold, because their calorie balance system is stable at a normal level for them.

Earlier, I mentioned a study by Jules Hirsch and his colleagues at Rockefeller University. They studied a group of people who were overweight and had succeeded in lowering their body weight to the accepted normal range. They found that when their body weight was within the so-called normal range, they needed 25 percent fewer calories to maintain their body weight than people of the same weight who had never been obese. This is another characteristic of genetic obesity, a need to severely limit the calorie intake to avoid regaining the weight that has been lost.

Hirsch and colleagues believe that when a person stays below his or her normal weight by severe dietary restrictions, that causes a condition similar to anorexia nervosa, a severe form of undernutrition. They found that these people had very tiny fat cells. It may be that the number of cells and their size, as examined from a fat biopsy under a microscope, will provide a good clue as to who is overweight for genetic reasons and who is not. The individuals in the Hirsch study exhibited other evidences of undernutrition, including loss of normal menstrual periods, low blood pressure and slow heart rates. They exhibited some of the same changes caused by undernutrition in the young men in the Minnesota experiment.

How can you manage genetic obesity? The best approach is probably not to try. Work with nature not against it. Some people, who are overweight for genetic reasons, also have extra fat from overeating and from underactivity. These aspects of their problem can be managed by a diet that provides a normal number of calories and a sensible level of physical activity. The body will adjust to its proper level if you provide the right environment for it, and let nature take its course.

It is important that individuals who are overweight because of genes have an adequate exercise program. Often, in part because of being overweight, these people are not as active as they should be. Another problem is that those with a lot of extra pounds may find it difficult to engage in many forms of exercise. Even walking to eliminate calories may prove difficult for those who have arthritis. For people who are overweight and have arthritis, a stationary bicycle is a real help. Many people prefer to use a stationary bicycle and to stay indoors while exercising, although, they can certainly cycle outdoors if they choose. Of course, inclement weather may make cycling outdoors difficult. A bicycle takes some of the weight off the knees and hips, which makes it possible to exercise with less difficulty. Overweight individuals also do well to exercise in water. Swimming is an excellent exercise to stimulate your calorie-loss mechanism, and the growth of your active energy tissues. It will not be as useful to strengthen bones or prevent osteoporosis, simply because it eliminates the effects of the body's weight on the skeleton.

A very real factor in preventing people with overweight problems from exercising is their self-consciousness. If they have to expose their bodies, they may avoid exercise. You see this in people who do not want to go swimming in public places. They will often tell you, "I wouldn't be caught dead in a bathing suit." Yes, this is a hang-up on the part of the overweight individual, but it develops because of society's attitude about overweight people. It is a reaction to discrimination.

Middle-Aged Spread

Both men and women hate to see their youthful figures undergoing changes as they approach middle-age. In a society that places a premium on youth, this is a depressing development. What really happens? Remember that your brain has all the controls to regulate how fat you are. It can stimulate you to eat more. It can turn your metabolic furnaces up or down, and it can turn your heat-loss mechanism on or off. Remember, also, that genes have a major influence on how much you should weigh. It doesn't take much imagination to realize that your brain determines what you should weight at each phase of your life. Your brain has a biological script for your life. The script contains the timetable for when your first teeth will erupt, when you will lose your baby teeth and gain your permanent teeth and when puberty will begin. It contains the rhythm cycle that controls a female's menstrual cycle. It controls the onset of the menopause. It controls when and if your body will get fatter. Stop and think for a minute about what happens at puberty to the female. She starts developing fat deposits that she did not have before. Those secondary sexual characteristics are normal, and the timing of their development is determined by the brain.

Many women think that middle-aged spread is caused by the menopause. That may be a factor in some cases as the two ovarian hormones, estrogen and progesterone, have a feedback mechanism with brain chemicals, called neurotransmitters that can play a role in controlling body fat. But contrary to popular belief, middle-aged weight gain is usually not because of a lack of ovarian hormones. People tend to explain events on a cause and effect basis. The thought is that a woman enters the menopause and, because of ovarian failure, she gets fat, a cause and effect relationship. But the real truth is that the brain can trigger both the menopause and the change in body weight. It doesn't have to do both. Some women gain weight before the menopause. Those who gain weight with or after the menopause usually remain overweight, even if they have hormone replacement therapy. You can replace the ovarian hormones that have decreased, but you can't stop that script inside the brain. Another indicator of the independent relationship of the menopause and gaining weight is that many women go through the menopause and do not gain weight, even though they do not decrease their calorie intake or increase their level of physical activity. These are the lucky women whose genetic program does not call for them to gain weight, and they may never gain weight throughout their lives.

It is often said that the thermostat in the brain is reset at the time of the menopause, and that is why a woman gains weight. In fact, the thermostat may be reset. Many postmenopausal women do notice that their body temperature is lower than it used to be. That may be part of the mechanisms triggered by the brain to enhance weight gain. But the brain has all the various controls at its disposal to ensure that you weigh within the range predetermined by your genetic script, for your age.

There are other factors that contribute to the middle-aged spread in some people. By that time in life, they may become physically less active. That can also mean that they do not do as many things that load the muscles or make them work against resistance. It is a time when the amount of muscle can decrease. A decrease in muscle weight means the body will require fewer calories. If the calorie intake stays the same, a person will increase his or her body fat. Remember the example of Magnus Levy.

What can you do to avoid middle-aged spread? You need to be sure the increased weight is not the result of your having slipped into an overeating-overweight or underactive-overweight pattern. A balanced diet and a sensible exercise program is as far as you should go. Again, it's not wise to fight your body.

The Yo-Yo Phenomenon

The truth is that most people who lose body weight regain it. That is not too surprising when you consider that the brain and genetic system has set a weight range for most people. The result is that you can fight your body and win the battle, but your body wins the war. You have already seen how many different ways the body has of fighting back when you try to trim it down. You don't always have to go back to the same lifestyle you had before to regain weight, either. Just relax the more strict measures, return to a normal living pattern with a reasonable diet, and presto, your body snaps up those extra calories and replenishes your fat cells. Only when you have regained your former weight is your body satisfied. When you consider your entire calorie balance system, you can see why a short interval of negative calorie balance might not have much of an effect.

Exercise is the best way we know to drive your metabolic system to eliminate calories from the body. The drawback is that as you lose calories, your brain will stimulate you to consume more calories to make up for the loss. Exercise is often a great stimulus to the appetite. It is necessary to control your calorie intake while you are increasing your physical activity, or you will be back where your brain wants you to be in short order.

The yo-yo effect in a person who is heavy by normal standards usually means that he or she has inherited a tendency to weigh that amount, and after each effort to lose weight, the brain controls the system to return the body weight to normal. Of course, there are some individuals who simply never learned to eat properly and return to consuming foods excessively rich in calories, or stop being active.

There is an important point to remember about the yo-yo reaction to losing weight. The initial loss in many of these cases is induced by a severe restriction of calories. Remember that the first few days of a total fast is when the body loses important body protein, while it is converting to using fat stores for energy. If a person goes on a severely restricted diet regularly, or fasts one day a week, that person will lose more body protein each time this occurs. Each time the metabolic furnace is decreased in its capacity, and each time this makes it more difficult to lose weight in the future.

When You Can't Lose Weight

The person who has really tried to lose weight and can't is often discouraged. This happens most often to a small, stocky woman. Judging from the letters I get, these women may actually stay on diets of fewer than 800 calories a day, while also following a regular exercise program. Some would doubt their story, but I believe them. What can be done about such a problem?

The first thing is to be sure there is no medical problem causing the difficulty, such as low thyroid function. If everything is normal, the next thing is to find out what the energy requirements really are. To do this, I still think the best measurement is to find out how much oxygen is used under near-basal conditions, then calculate how many calories are needed each day just for the near-basal requirements. If the test shows that the near-basal calorie requirement is 1,500 calories, that person probably is not staying on an 800-calorie diet. When the energy requirements, calculated from oxygen consumption, are really low, the metabolic furnace may have been turned down for some reason, such as a medical condition, or that person has a very small fat-free body weight.

In the latter case, the approach is not to decrease the calories even more. It is better to try to develop the metabolically-active fat-free body weight. That means more exercise. It may even mean easing up on the calorie restriction while stressing exercise. Since such a person needs to build metabolically-active tissue, the exercise should be directed toward muscle-building. A sensible muscle-building program over a period of many months, properly planned and carried out along the lines known to actually stimulate muscle development, may be the best thing that can be done. All of the things you would do for a bodybuilder need to be considered. That means enough good quality protein to support muscle development.

If that fails, it is important to accept the fact that the body fat is probably hereditary, and that person's apparent extra body fat is the way he or she is supposed to be.

Summary 14

1. Overeating-overweight people are overweight simply because they consume too many calories. Dietary restriction is the best approach to this problem.
2. Underactive-overweight people may consume a normal number of calories but are overweight because of lack of physical activity. These people do better by gradually increasing their level of physical activity.
3. Genetic obesity is the problem of being overweight by usual standards because a person inherits the characteristics to weigh that much and the body makes every effort to maintain that standard. Often these people do not respond well to either calorie restriction or increased physical activity or both. With heroic efforts they can lose weight, but that is not always good for their health.
4. The middle-aged spread is often a normal form of weight gain that is also genetic. A person inherits a script for different stages of

life and at the middle-aged stage that script often calls for an increased amount of body fat.

5. The yo-yo body weight phenomenon with repeated short periods of inadequate nutrition is the most likely to cause a person to lose essential body protein.

6. People who are genetically intended to be "overweight" should probably accept their characteristic in the same way we accept whether we are short or tall, unless there is a real medical indication that requires loss of body fat.

Chapter 15

Girth Control

DEAR DR. LAMB: Do men have pot bellies more than women? My husband has developed one since retirement, yet his weight remains the same as it has been for years—which is not high. Could one or two beers a day and not exercising contribute to this? He has never done much exercise so I doubt this would be a factor now. He doesn't gain weight any place else. This belly is very firm, not flabby—almost like being pregnant in the way it looks and feels.

Any exercise routine would have to be quite limited for him because he does have only 50 percent of his breathing capacity and has a touch of emphysema. He did quit smoking about six years ago, thank God. Lately he has started exercising on a rowing machine. He is 69.

How to avoid the big middle is often one challenge of the middle-aged spread, but girth control can be a problem at any age. Men are more prone to this problem earlier in life than women. It now seems apparent that the excess fat around the middle is related to the nature of the fat cells themselves. In people who have a tendency to develop fat over the abdomen, there is an increased number of fat cells that have alpha$_2$ receptors. It is hard to get fat cells with these receptors to give up their fat. They load fat easily, in preference to other fat cells, and are the last to give it up. That is why a person can lose fat in other areas of the body, but not there. It is also why spot reducing doesn't work.

You have to be careful in evaluating what causes an enlarged abdomen. Girth control is not always a matter of fat deposits. The classic example is that of a woman being pregnant. In other instances there may be enlargement of organs—such as the liver or the spleen—or even a tumor inside the abdomen. In still other cases there may be an accumulation of excess fluid inside the abdomen, for example in response to liver disease. Notice that his wife describes her husband's abdomen as firm and doesn't mention a roll of fat—the familiar spare tire. That raises my suspicion that there may be something else other than "belly fat" involved. If he has had a habit of drinking a lot for a long time, you have to wonder if he has liver disease. But she does say he has emphysema. In this condition the lungs are overinflated and that pushes the diaphragm down. That makes the abdominal cavity shorter and leaves only one place for the abdominal organs to go—out. And that means enlargement of the abdominal girth. Of course, it could be fat. Incidentally he could do the most important exercise for flattening his stomach without very much physical effort, the voluntary contractions, which I'll explain later.

Women can also have an excess number of alpha$_2$ fat cells over the abdomen. More characteristically they have excess fat over the thighs and buttocks which this lady writes about.

DEAR DR. LAMB: I am 43 years old, 5 feet 2 and weigh 180 pounds. My problem is big legs and abdomen. I have had three children. One was stillborn and had to be pulled out. This left my abdominal muscles weak. At my age I will soon be going through the menopause. I was told that once a woman stopped her periods, even if you lose weight, you would keep all the flab. If I go on a 1,000 calorie diet and do daily exercises, can this stomach be pulled in? Once I did this and lost weight, but I was younger then. I'm also heavy busted. Is there an exercise along with the diet to help me?

At 5 feet 2 and weighing 180 pounds it is a safe conclusion that this lady has more than an enlarged abdomen. She can be certain that she has a lot of fat inside the abdomen too. She probably needs a lot of help to eliminate general obesity. It is surprising how few people seem to realize that they accumulate fat inside the body too. You can't lose your abdominal girth without eliminating the fat inside the body. But exercise and calorie restriction is not always the answer as is apparent from this lady's letter.

DEAR DR. LAMB: I am 40 years old and in reasonably good health. I'm 5 feet 5 and weigh 135 pounds. My problem is I have always had a pot belly. Even during high school when I was a cheerleader and did exercises constantly, including sit-ups, I had a pot belly.

My husband insists that I could get it off with the proper exercise, but I know better. I have weighed 118 before, was in perfect shape and still had it.

What can I do to eliminate this unwanted pot?

Accepting this lady's story as she tells it strongly suggests that she will not be successful with exercises and a diet. She is most likely one of those individuals who have an excess number of the special fat cells that do not reduce. She was probably born with these. These people can benefit some from a diet and exercise program, but in the last analysis, many of these individuals are the very ones who really need surgical removal of fat cells. I'll say more about that later.

Some investigators think these women are more prone to heart disease than women who do not have this type of fat distribution. As I mentioned before, women more often have an excess of alpha$_2$ fat cells over the buttocks and thighs and men are prone to the abdominal fat cells.

Get the Fat Out

In most cases there is about as much fat inside the abdomen as there is outside beneath the skin. There is one structure inside the abdomen that is like a great sheet of plastic wrapping tissue, called the *omentum*. It hangs from the curved outer edge of the stomach like a great apron, and covers the abdominal organs. It is a good place for fat to accumulate. In people who have a very fat abdomen, this can be a huge layer of fat lying between the abdominal muscular wall and the abdominal organs. In cases of extreme obesity, this large apron has been removed by surgery. This does not mean I am advocating surgery to remove the fat inside your abdomen. It is important, though, for you to realize that a major factor in girth control is the fat *inside the abdomen*, as well as the fat outside, under your skin. In some situations the fat inside the abdomen, in the omentum, and outside under the skin results in a really large abdomen as described by this man's letter.

DEAR DR. LAMB: Please identify the apron-like membrane called the "omentum" that you mentioned in your column. You mention that surgeons have to use a "block-and-tackle" device to lift the huge mass of fat in obese people needing abdominal surgery.

I have seen a few short, very obese women, while walking, kick something under their skirts. I thought at first it was a breeze as they came through the revolving door, but once into the building, it happened over and over again — this sudden "thrust" or billowing out" like a ball. I could not believe my eyes.

Is this the omentum or apron you referred to? Did it just grow and grow and all that flab stretch all the way down to the knees, like rising bread dough overflowing a bread pan? Can the flab be cut off or suctioned off?

Of course you cannot see the omentum since it is inside the abdominal cavity. But some very obese women do have such a large layer of abdominal fat that it will hang down below the pubic area, like a huge apron. These people need lots of medical supervision to solve their problem. And I must say, we really don't know what this man saw. Another reader suggested he was seeing the take from a shop-lifting spree.

There are two goals in shrinking that pot. One is to eliminate the fat, and the other is to tighten up the muscles. No matter how tight you make your muscles, you will not be able to have a flat stomach without getting the fat out of your abdominal cavity, as well as from under your skin. Think of your abdomen as a large plastic bag filled with water. You can squeeze it, pound it, and exert pressure on it in any way you wish, but it will not get smaller unless you break the plastic bag. That fat inside your abdomen behaves in the same way. You could have a set of abdominals that Arnold Schwarzenegger would be proud of, but if you have fat inside the abdomen, you will not have a flat stomach. A person who wants to reduce his or her stomach will need to follow a program that controls the calorie balance and eliminates excess pounds of fat. Make no mistake about it, though, the effort to improve your appearance by losing that fat may not be the right thing for you to do. Just like any other type of overweight problem, you have to consider what is causing it. If you were meant to be that way, inducing a negative calorie balance may not be the right answer.

Three Types of Exercises

Naturally I got a lot of letters asking about exercises to flatten the stomach. People are confused about what to expect from the exercises used for this purpose. This is a typical query.

> DEAR DR. LAMB: I am interested in knowing which of the following is the most effective exercise to flatten the stomach: walking, riding a bicycle, or doing leg lifts and sit-ups.

The real answer is none of the above. All of these can help to some degree but none are the most important exercise. Walking on level ground does not use your abdominal muscles at all, just those of your legs. Riding a bicycle is the same. Most leg lifts don't exercise the abdominal muscles either and sit-ups must be done properly and they only affect your two long muscles that stretch from your rib cage to your pubic bone on each side of your navel. These muscles are not the most important ones to keep you from having a relaxed and large abdomen. The really important ones are your flat abdominal muscles that are like sheets of muscle around the sides of the abdomen and these are strengthened by doing voluntary contractions, which you can do without bending your torso at all—in a chair, in bed or standing.

In addition, you need to do exercises that improve the posture. That includes straightening the spine so you will stand up properly.

Despite these seemingly negative comments the exercises you can do to strengthen your trunk muscles may be very helpful, even though they may not produce all the results that you would like.

The Sit-Up

There are many versions of doing sit-up exercises. To develop strong abdominal muscles, you must contract them against resistance. During a sit-up you are using your body weight as the resistance. Sit-up exercises are primarily for the upper abdomen. They use the rectus abdominis, those two big muscles on each side of your navel that I mentioned. These muscles do only one thing, pull your chest, or tip of your breast bone, closer to your pubic bone. You can lie flat on the floor with your knees bent and then raise your head and shoulders off the floor. About three fourths of the way off the floor is the limit of the exercise that really loads these two muscles. Thereafter, you are using muscles that help to bend the hip toward the abdomen, to close the hip angle. That means it is not really necessary to lean all the way forward to your knees.

You should hold the sit-up for just a few seconds, then relax and return to the beginning position. Remember the principles of strength training. It will not strengthen your muscles to do 50 or 60 sit-ups. Two or three sets of 10 sit-ups each, about every other day, will do as much as you can expect from sit-ups. If you want to develop endurance, you can do more, but don't expect too much. Originally, you may want to restrict your effort to no more than two sets of 10 sit-ups. Allow your muscles to get a little stronger before you try to go for endurance.

At the beginning, you may not be able to do 10 sit-ups. Put your hands on your bent knees and help pull yourself up. As you gain strength in your abdominal muscles, you will need less and less help with your hands.

How can you load your abdominal muscle more? Don't try it until you can do the two sets of 10-sit ups easily, without hands and without fatigue. Then, you may find doing them on a slant board will help. You can even use resistance machines to work against. A simple way to do sit-ups and get about the maximum load from your own body is to lie on the floor and put your feet on a couch or chair. Do this so your knees are bent at nearly a right angle. Now do the regular sit-ups. These more stressful sit-ups are not for the beginner. Use a few of the simple ones to start with and don't overdo it to the point that you have sore abdominal muscles.

It is important to avoid doing sit-ups with your knees straight and your legs stretched straight out on the floor. When you do a sit-up in that position, you are using the muscles that help bend your hips more than exercising the abdominal muscles.

You also have oblique muscles that are laced across your abdomen. You can work these some by modifying your sit-up exercises. Start your sit-up by raising your left shoulder off the floor and toward your right knee. Relax, and then lift your right shoulder off the floor and toward your left knee. Ten of each, a rest, then repeating the 10 of each, is usually adequate.

Easy With the Leg Lifts

Despite what many people think, leg-lifts do almost nothing to strengthen the abdominal muscles. What little benefit a person gets is really from tensing the abdominal muscles while lifting the legs and you can do that better with the voluntary contractions which I will discuss. The reason the leg-lifts do almost nothing is that when you bend the thigh toward the abdomen to lift the feet off the floor you contract muscles that are attached to the femur (thigh bone) at one end and to the spine at the other end. These muscles are not part of the abdominal wall at all. Since leg-lifts do not contract the abdominal muscles, it is little wonder that they don't accomplish much in flattening your abdomen.

If you choose to do them, remember that they can actually injure your back if you do them too vigorously or strain too much. Individuals with back complaints should not do these exercises without asking their doctor about them first. The easiest way to do them is to lie flat on the floor with your knees bent. Then raise your bent knees up toward your chest. Now tighten your abdominal muscles and straighten your knees, then bend your knees as you bring your feet back to the original position.

Voluntary Contractions Safe

The voluntary contractions of your abdominal muscles are the most important exercises to flatten your abdomen. While you are seated, put your fingers on the sides of your abdomen, just below your ribs. Now pull your stomach in and you should feel these muscles. There are three flat muscles layered one on top of the other that contract to pull your abdominal girth in. Basically they are attached to the ribs at the front of your abdomen, wrap around your trunk and attach to your spine. They act like a belt or girdle from the top to the bottom of your abdomen. The edge of these three muscles ends in a tough fibrous sheath that wraps around the two rectus muscles you use when you do sit-ups. These flat muscles are the ones you push with when you are having a bowel movement. They are the ones you contract when you pull your abdomen in, "sucking in your gut," as the less dignified phrase puts it. They are the one's that normally hold in your girth. You

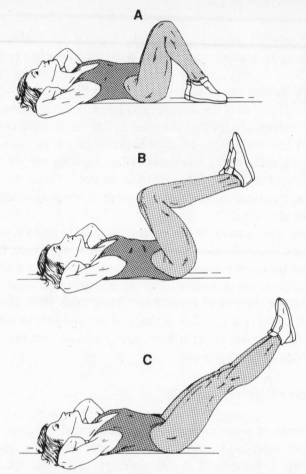

Leg-lifts can hurt your back. If you do them, start with the knees bent. When you straighten your knees from **B** to **C**, contract (pull in) your abdominal muscles to provide support. That voluntary contraction of the abdominal muscles is the part that is the most helpful.

do not go around contracting your rectus abdominis muscle you use in sit-ups.

You can also strengthen these flat abdominal muscles by simply contracting them voluntarily. While lying on the floor, with the knees bent, simply pull in and contract the abdominal muscles as forceably

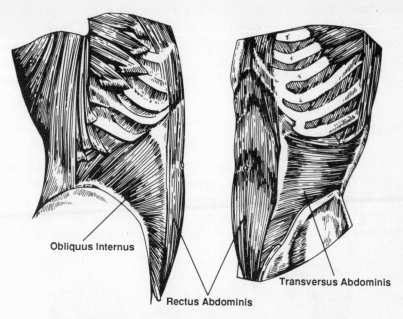

Obliquus Internus

Transversus Abdominis

Rectus Abdominis

The three flat muscles at the sides of the rectus abdominis are the important muscles that hold your abdomen in. They work like a belt or girdle. When they contract, they pull in the abdomen, but contracting the rectus abdominis pulls the tip of the sternum toward your pubic arch. The three flat muscles are the obliquus externus, obliquus internus, and the transversus abdominis. Note they attach to the sides of the large rectus abdominis muscles. The obliquus externus is not pictured, but is the muscle layer just outside the obliquus internus and its muscle fibers are perpendicular to those of the obliquus internus. The transversus abdominis is the inner layer of the three flat muscles. The best and only way to exercise these flat muscles is by voluntary contractions or tensing (pulling in) and relaxing the abdominal wall. They are not affected by either sit-ups or leg-lifts unless you consciously contract and relax them at the same time.

as you can. Hold the position to the count of five then relax. Repeat 10 times, relax a few minutes, then do a second set of 10. You can do these same exercises while sitting. That makes it perfect for the person who has to sit. You can also see why the man who had emphysema and could do little exercise could do this type of exercise. There is little danger in hurting your back or anything else with this exercise, as you are not putting any strain on the back. But you can get sore abdominal muscles from overdoing it, just as you can from overdoing any exercise.

Straighten the Back

Your posture has a lot to do with how much your abdomen protrudes. That is why exercises to strengthen your back muscles can help you. Think of your spine as a large bow, and the abdominal muscles as a string between each end of the bow. As you bend the bow, the string becomes slack. In the same way, if you bend your spine forward, your

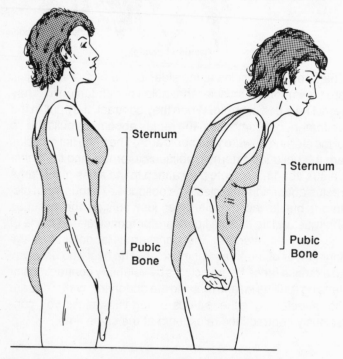

When you slump or bend forward, you lose the normal lumbar curve in the small of the back and the sternum is closer to the pubic bone. This causes the abdominal wall to expand outward.

abdominal muscles will be slack. Note, that as you bend over to pick up something from the floor, your abdomen literally falls outward, unless you consciously pull it in. The two ends of the bow, so to speak, are the bottom of the rib cage and the pubic bone, where the large, paired rectus abdominis muscles attach. If you bend in a way to bring your rib cage closer to your pubic bone, it is like bending the bow, and it decreases tension on your abdominal muscles. Good posture should include keeping your spine erect enough to spread the distance between your ribs and the pubic bone. To do that, you need to maintain the normal arch in the spine in the small of your back, between your ribs and your buttocks. That often requires strengthening the muscles in the small of your back, the lumbar area.

The best way to strengthen these is to simply sit on the floor on your feet, with your knees bent. Bend forward, as if to touch your forehead on the floor. Now consciously raise your head and upper body by

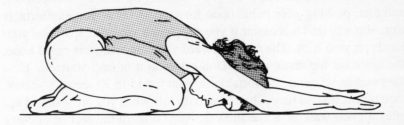

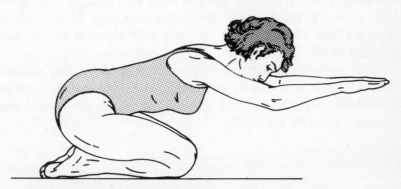

Bending forward when on your knees, then raising the upper body while arcing the back, uses the back muscles.

contracting the muscles in your back. Don't just bend your hip muscles to change your position, but use those spinal muscles. Arch your back as much as it is comfortable for you to do without straining. When you first start these exercises, you can put your hands on your knees to support yourself and help yourself as you raise your upper body.

You may also benefit by strengthening the muscles in your upper back that help to lift your shoulders up and back. You want to use exercises that help to improve your ability to open your spine, and avoid the curled fetal position.

Open Your Hip Angle

One of the more neglected points in maintaining good posture is keeping the hip angle open. Try it by standing up as straight as possible and then pushing your pubic bone forward as far as you comfortably can. You will find it is easier if you stand with your feet apart and your hands on your hips. The more forward you can push your pubic bone, the more the hip angle opens. Don't overdo it or hurt yourself. Hold the position which is comfortable for you for 15 to 30 seconds. Relax, then repeat several times. It is best to do this when you are warmed up, after a good walk or a hot shower. As you learn the feel of opening your hip angle, you may want to do it while standing in a doorway with one hand on each side of the door jamb. The whole point is to loosen up your hip joint, so you can stand with your pubic bone forward enough to provide good support for your body. As you will notice, it affects the whole way you hold your abdomen and, in turn, affects your girth.

Other exercises to strengthen your trunk muscles, and maintain their full range of motion by stretching, are helpful, but these are the main ones. they will go a long way toward helping you control your girth and avoid the big middle.

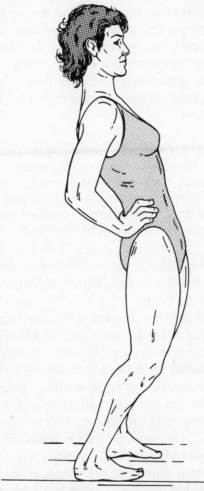

Opening the hip angle is just the opposite of bending forward at the hips. It helps to stretch muscles and improve posture. The upright posture that avoids closing the hip angle helps hold the abdominal wall in.

Fat Suction and Abdominal Fat

I mentioned earlier that one way to get rid of those special fat cells that hold fat forever is to cut them out. That has been done for years. There is a counterpart to this in the rat experiments I mentioned earlier, where half of the littermates had part of their fat tissue removed and they stopped getting fat in those areas. Formerly, to remove these persistent fat areas, rather large incisions were required. Today, a technique called liposuction has changed that. That is the procedure this lady is asking about.

> DEAR DR. LAMB: I saw on TV that fat could be sucked out of parts of your body. I need this done to my stomach. I'm 60 years old and look nine months pregnant. I was somewhat overweight and lost a lot of weight, but not any from my stomach. In fact, I think my stomach looks larger now. This is doing something to my marriage. My husband will not take me out anymore. Can this fat be eliminated?

This procedure does literally suck out fat from under your skin. It will eliminate love handles and spare tires. It is also used in other places, such as over the thighs.

A very small incision is made and a flexible suction probe is guided under the skin to the fat areas and the fat cells are simply sucked out. The technique has been improved greatly since it was first introduced. Smaller, more flexible probes are important. They cannot remove large amounts of fat at one time. There is always a danger that removing too much fat will cause a person to go into shock. Obviously you can't use this method to remove fat from inside the abdomen. It removes only fat between the skin and the muscular wall. I would add a note of caution to be sure that you see a physician who is well trained in this technique and used to handling problems related to surgery of the skin and fat. A plastic surgeon trained in these techniques is a good choice.

Summary 15

1. There are many different causes for a large abdomen besides fat deposits. That includes pregnancy, enlarged organs, tumors and fluid.

2. People with large amounts of abdominal fat usually have increased numbers of the special fat cells that retain fat in that location.
3. Men are more prone to abdominal obesity than women, but it can occur in both sexes. Women are more prone to excess fat over the thighs and buttocks.
4. There is some evidence that individuals with a large amount of abdominal fat are more likely to have a heart attack than those who do not.
5. A major portion of the fat deposits that cause abdominal obesity are inside the abdomen. It is essential to lose this fat to flatten the stomach. That is why weight control measures are a necessary part of flattening an abdomen enlarged with fat.
6. Despite the popularity of sit-ups and leg-lifts, the best exercises to strengthen your abdomen are the voluntary contractions of the abdominal muscles—pulling your abdominal muscles in and holding the contraction, followed by relaxation and repetitions.
7. Exercises to strengthen the back in order to maintain good posture with the chest held up are important.
8. Surgical removal of fat, which can be liposuction, is a good way to remove those hard-to-eliminate fat deposits such as love handles and a spare tire.

Chapter 16

Medical Causes for Overweight

There is still a lot of confusion over whether being overweight causes disease or whether being overweight is a manifestation of an underlying disease. The truth is that both probably happen. It is like the story of rats and mice. Some strains have genes that cause them to get fat on a perfectly normal diet. But rats that do not have these genetic defects and are perfectly normal can get fat too, from consuming high calorie foods that provide more calories than the rat can use. Some people who are overweight because of consuming too many calories and not being physically active develop problems of high blood pressure and high total cholesterol levels in response to their habits. Others have a genetic makeup that causes a number of abnormalities, such as a high total cholesterol, high blood pressure and even a high blood glucose level as well as a tendency to be overweight. And even if a disease is caused by genetic factors, such as a high total cholesterol level that can be found in families, elimination of excess body fat often proves helpful.

People often search for a reason to explain why they have unwanted body fat. That is particularly true if they have stayed on a restricted diet, and have been reasonably active, but still remain overweight. They usually wonder if they have a medical problem. There are many well-defined medical disorders that will cause a person to be overweight, but they are seldom the cause for the weight problems most people have. Rather, most weight problems are related to an inherited tendency to be "overweight," or from consuming too many calorie-rich foods or not maintaining enough physical activity. I include the changes with different phases of life in a life script as part of a person's inherited tendency.

Overweight and Hypothyroid

Of all the various medical conditions people think they may have as a cause for being overweight, low thyroid function is high on the list. That feeling is reinforced because thyroid has been prescribed for many patients trying to lose weight. But unless a person actually does have a hypothyroid condition, that is not helpful. There are a few people who are overweight because of low thyroid function, however; the disorder only occurs in about 1.4 percent of adult females in the United States, and only in 0.1 percent of adult males. Obviously, a low thyroid condition is far less common than being overweight. Not all people with a hypothyroid condition are grossly overweight. Usually, they have only a modest weight gain, of as little as 10 pounds. The severe, advanced state of hypothyroidism is called *myxedema*. It may result in the retention of a mucus-like complex sugar that causes local retention of water and may result in swelling.

People who have hypothyroid conditions have symptoms of low metabolic activity. Remember that thyroid hormone stimulates the metabolic action of body cells. When there is not enough thyroid hormone, or the inactive reverse triiodothyronine (rT_3) is formed, this activity slows down and the body produces less heat. The skin is cold, since it doesn't need to be so active in eliminating calories of heat. It is not surprising that people with a low thyroid condition complain of cold intolerance. They feel cold because there is so little blood flowing through the skin. In addition, they may complain of fatigue. They have little energy, because their cells are not releasing a lot of energy. If you measured their oxygen consumption, as was once a standing ritual in evaluating a person for thyroid function, you would find they had a decreased oxygen utilization. The relationship between calorie use, heat produced and oxygen utilization does apply. Because of the decreased need for oxygen, the heart beats slowly and the amount of blood it pumps is decreased.

These people do not have a large appetite. They do not need a lot of food to sustain their low metabolic level. In some manner, the brain senses this and that is why they are not stimulated to eat much. That is also why they are usually not grossly overweight. They present the picture of a person whose entire calorie balance system has been lowered, including the number of calories consumed, the number of calories released by their metabolic furnace and the number of calories eliminated through the skin. Of course, they have other symptoms as well.

A person who is hypothyroid is correctly treated by replacing the needed thyroid hormone. That will usually reverse all of these symptoms, cause the cells to increase their metabolism and use more oxygen, release more heat, increase blood flow through the skin, improve the sense of warmth and increase the person's level of energy. *But, if a person is not hypothyroid, giving him or her thyroid hormone will not correct the overweight condition.*

Your thyroid gland has a wonderful, built-in stabilizing mechanism. It releases a normal amount of thyroid hormone to maintain your metabolic functions at the right level, and to facilitate other bodily functions. If you take thyroid hormone, the gland simply stops producing as much. As you increase the amount of thyroid you take, the gland eventually stops producing thyroid hormone at all, and you are back where you started in terms of the amount of thyroid hormone in your body. If you persist, and take even more thyroid hormone than your gland normally produces, then you start causing a hyperthyroid condition, which has the opposite effects of a low thyroid condition. It is not healthy to be hyperthyroid, and it causes its own symptoms.

It is instructive in understanding your calorie balance system, though, to see what happens to a person with an overactive thyroid condition. The cells are stimulated to an increased level of metabolism, so they use a lot more foodstuffs. That will cause the body to mobilize and use the existing fat stores. The victim will eat and eat and eat. The brain is stimulating the appetite to provide enough fuel for that metabolic furnace, to prevent using the body tissues to supply it. Such a high level of metabolism uses a lot of oxygen. That requires the heart to work harder, and the heart rate is usually fast. The metabolic activity also releases a lot of heat. That heat must be eliminated through the skin, so hyperthyroid people complain of being hot. Their skin is moist, while the skin of a patient with a hypothyroid condition is dry and cold. As the body heat rises, the full effects of the air-conditioning effort of the skin are turned on by the brain. A patient with a very active thyroid may be resting quietly in a cool room, the body thin and lightly clothed, but sweat may be pouring off the skin.

All of these evidences of an overactive metabolic system are eliminated by correcting the overactive thyroid state.

Because the thyroid gland in a normal person just shuts down when he or she is given thyroid hormone, it is clear that the small doses sometimes used to try to help people lose weight are useless. If you take 60 mg of thyroid hormone, the thyroid gland just puts out 60 mg less. Any benefits a person may think he gets from taking small amounts of thyroid are purely psychological, and not because of the thyroid hormone's action.

Overweight Because of Hypoglycemia

Hypoglycemia (low blood sugar) and hypothyroidism are probably the two most common medical conditions people suspect of causing their excess weight. Usually neither is the cause. Hypoglycemia has been a popular diagnosis in both lean and overweight individuals, but the diagnosis is often wrong. The public has been caught up in the selling of "low blood sugar" as a cause for many not well defined symptoms. But a careful review of the situation by authorities in the field has led the American Medical Association to warn physicians about overdiagnosing hypoglycemia and they have set guide lines to follow. Such a diagnosis should never be made unless a person has the typical symptoms of hypoglycemia at the same time a blood test shows that the blood level of glucose is really low. A low blood glucose level without symptoms is not an adequate basis for a diagnosis. Neither are symptoms, without establishing that the blood glucose level is low at the time they occur. The public perception of hypoglycemia is far different from the medical facts. That is what causes the confusion expressed by this lady's letter.

DEAR DR. LAMB: My doctor says I don't have hypoglycemia. I don't think he believes there is such an ailment. I need to lose about 15 pounds. When I try to cut down, I get ravenously hungry. Sometimes I tremble and my hands shake. I eat with both hands until this stops. My diet is then ruined again.

I eat healthy foods and only 1,200 to 1,400 calories when I cut down. When I drink coffee on an empty stomach I also have to eat something or I become shaky and kind of nauseated.

My doctor did a four-hour test for hypoglycemia and said I was OK.

I'm a 63-year-old woman. Do you have any idea what will help me to lose these ugly pounds?

The symptoms this woman is describing are most likely caused by the release of adrenaline, our stress hormone. Hypoglycemia causes the body to release adrenaline. The adrenaline causes the liver to mobilize glycogen to raise the blood glucose. The catch is that anxiety and stress can also cause a release of adrenaline. Regardless of what causes the release of the adrenaline, the end results are the same. Consequently, a lot of people who have anxiety get an unwarranted diagnosis of hypoglycemia. This woman's comments about coffee are interesting, because the caffeine in coffee enhances the adrenaline reaction whether the adrenaline is released because of stress or from hypoglycemia.

Hypoglycemia is equated to an increased amount of insulin. It is true that the rare condition of an increased production of insulin will stimulate the storage of fat. Insulin has three actions related to one's becoming overweight. It is important for the chemical reactions that are necessary to form fat. It is important in the storage and in preventing the release of fat from fat cells. And it lowers the blood glucose, which in turn stimulates the appetite, resulting in overeating.

I have always remembered the animal caretaker for the pharmacology department when I was in medical school. He was tall and thin, but he had not always been that way. In earlier days, Archie was very fat. He had medical problems, and the faculty was hard pressed to know what was wrong. However, they did know that he ate a lot. Finally, it was discovered that he had a tumor of the islets of Langerhans, in the pancreas, which was pouring out insulin. He was responding to the effects of insulin by overeating, forming fat, then storing and retaining fat. The tumor was removed, and the excess insulin production stopped. His appetite returned to normal. His body got rid of the large excess amount of body fat, and when I knew him, he was skinny. It didn't take a special diet to get rid of his excess fat. His body adjusted itself when the tumor was removed.

Today, there are still a lot of overweight people who think they have, or have been told they have, reactive hypoglycemia. That is a lot different from the islet cell tumor. The theory is that when these people eat sweets or starches, their blood glucose rises, which in turn causes the islets of Langerhans to pour out insulin. It overdoes this, and the blood glucose falls to low levels, causing the symptoms of hypoglycemia. The insulin also is believed to stimulate the actions that lead to obesity. In fact, many of these people are overweight because they are anxious, and because they are anxious they form adrenaline. They have adrenaline symptoms from anxiety, not hypoglycemia. Unless there is a bona fide diagnosis of hypoglycemia, manipulating the diet in these individuals will do very little to correct their overweight condition. Why? Because hypoglycemia is not the cause of their being overweight in the first place.

Diabetic and Overweight

One of the confusing aspects of diabetes is that it can be associated with being either overweight or underweight. There is another interesting aspect: diabetes that starts in childhood is often caused by a viral disease, while diabetes that first starts in adult life is more often associated with a family history and has an inherited tendency. The diabetes that occurs first in childhood is often called juvenile diabetes and is now called type I insulin-dependent diabetes. The diabetes that first occurs in adult life used to be called adult-onset diabetes and is now referred to as type II or non-insulin dependent diabetes—even though type II diabetes may be severe enough to require insulin therapy. Evidently, these individuals with an inherited tendency are programmed to develop diabetes later in life. The overweight individual may only have an abnormal blood glucose level (abnormal glucose tolerance). If the abnormality in glucose metabolism progresses, it may become diabetes. Eventually, when the disease progresses until the diabetic is losing a lot of sugar in the urine, he will start losing weight. This person's letter is typical of the common case of the overweight diabetic.

> DEAR DR. LAMB: I was diagnosed as a diabetic and put on insulin four years ago. I was also told to lose weight. My physician says I may be able to get off the shots if I lose the required weight—in my case 45 pounds or more. I have tried losing this required weight only to gain back the few pounds I did lose. When I look on the drug store shelves there are all kinds of over-the-counter weight-loss pills, but they state, not to be used by people with high blood pressure, diabetes and other

medical problems. I am desperate to know if there is any kind of weight loss pills or medicine for diabetic and high blood pressure patients, as I suffer both. I exercise and diet, but my will power is shot.

It is interesting that the individual with just an abnormal glucose tolerance test, or mild diabetes not requiring insulin, will often develop normal glucose levels if he or she loses body fat. Not enough is really known about the interrelations to warrant speculation of what is involved. It could be that both increased body fatness and increased blood glucose are inherited traits in some individuals. In any case, one does not correct the blood glucose to correct the obesity. The opposite is true: correcting the excess weight problem will correct the high glucose levels. Even when oral medicines are given to lower the blood glucose level in these people, they do not lose weight. The glucose level may be normalized, but it doesn't affect the body fat stores. That is less often true in patients who require insulin, but some patients are successful in getting off insulin when they have a lot of weight to lose and do lose it.

Many of the over-the-counter pills for weight control do contain ingredients that may cause the blood pressure to rise and should not be used by people with high blood pressure. In fact, most of them should not be used by anybody, but I'll discuss them in the next chapter.

Eventually, the diabetic cannot utilize glucose from his carbohydrate foods or the glucose made from amino acids from protein. The weight loss that occurs is not from an increase in metabolism, but from a loss of calories, as glucose in the urine. In an effort to replace this loss, the brain will stimulate the appetite and the patient may eat a lot; however, he may not gain weight, but will continue to lose weight. This lady's letter describes the situation.

DEAR DR. LAMB: My husband is 46 years old and three years ago we found out he has sugar diabetes. He now controls it with two Diabinese daily. He follows a 2,400 calorie diet. We have also purchased a glucometer. His doctor wants him to check his blood glucose while fasting. His range is between 120 and 180, depending on the amount of work or exercise he has done.

What concerns me is his weight. Before getting diabetes, his weight was 160 to 165 pounds and he is 5 feet 11 inches tall. He is now 129 pounds. He feels good, but looks terrible. He has no body fat at all. His doctor doesn't seem to be concerned but did tell him not to lose any more.

My husband never did gain very easy, but now it is impossible. Every diabetic class we attended was on being overweight. Everyone was overweight but my husband. Is there any reason for my concern?

It is a safe bet that with a fasting glucose level of 180 it is much higher after eating. That also means it is high enough that he has probably been losing glucose in his urine. Which means calories lost through the kidneys. This man is probably not getting enough calories in his diet either. Note that his calorie intake is well below that normally recommended for a healthy person, and certainly inadequate for a person who is losing calories in his urine. That means he is probably a victim of undernutrition caused by his inadequate diet and made worse by his diabetes.

Rare Endocrine Disorders and Overweight

It is very rare for other endocrine disorders to actually be a cause for being overweight. Certain disorders of the ovaries may cause obesity, including polycystic ovaries (Stein Leventhal), or Turner's syndrome, a genetic defect. Hypogonadism in the male may be associated with being overweight. An excess secretion of corticosteroid hormones from the adrenal cortex may cause a peculiar form of obesity, as seen in Cushing's disease. As many as 90 percent of these rare individuals have a tumor of the pituitary gland under the brain that overstimulates the adrenal cortex. In about half of these individuals, the increased fat is over the trunk while the limbs are spared. The face is often moon-like and there are prominent fat deposits over the shoulders and back of the neck.

Medications and Overweight

Today, there is a vast array of medicines that affect brain chemistry. It is worth mentioning that some of them may cause weight gain, such as Periactin. These various medicines may act on serotonin and norepinephrine, both important brain chemicals that affect mood. Antidepressant medications and tranquilizers should also be suspect as possible causes for weight gain. These medicines may cause a weight gain by stimulating the appetite through mechanisms within the brain. The patient then eats far more calories than his metabolic system needs, and increased weight is the result. The person becomes overweight because of induced overeating.

There may be other mechanisms at work too. In some way these medicines may affect the brain's action in causing the loss of calories through heat loss. This is another area that needs further study.

It is worth noting that the large number of beta-blocker medicines—Inderal, Tenormin and others—used for heart disease, high blood pressure and other conditions may block the beta receptors of fat cells. That may prevent the mobilization of fat from these cells and contribute to obesity.

Summary 16

1. Some people develop diseases because they consume too many calories for their energy requirements. Others have inherited defects that cause both obesity and disease, such as high total cholesterol levels or diabetes.
2. A hypothyroid state will decrease metabolism, turning down your metabolic furnace and your energy requirements. But it is an uncommon cause for being overweight.
3. Except for the rare individual who is overweight because of low thyroid function, giving thyroid hormone to lose weight is not useful. If a person takes enough to cause a loss of weight, the results can be harmful.
4. Hypoglycemia, "low blood sugar," is rarely the cause for being overweight.
5. Real hypoglycemia, as caused by an insulin-producing tumor, will increase a person's appetite and may cause a significant overweight problem.
6. Anxiety and stress that result in an outpouring of adrenaline will produce many of the same symptoms ascribed to hypoglycemia.
7. Overweight adults with moderately high blood glucose levels will often have normal levels after losing excess body fat.
8. People who develop diabetes as an adult often have an inherited trait for diabetes and may also inherit the genes to become overweight. As a result, these diabetics are usually overweight.
9. In contrast, the person who develops diabetes in childhood requires insulin and is often underweight.

10. As a diabetic begins to lose glucose in the urine and fails to be able to use glucose for energy, he loses weight and may become a victim of undernutrition.
11. There are a number of rare endocrine disorders that cause a person to be overweight.
12. Some medications, particularly some of the antidepressants, may either stimulate the appetite or affect the heat-loss mechanism, or both, to cause significant weight gains.

Chapter 17

Help or Hazard

The search for a way to lose weight without effort, and to feel good, is never-ending. It includes drugs, surgery, and even special clothing, such as rubber sweat suits. It includes habits that people have incorporated into their lifestyles, such as drinking coffee and smoking cigarettes. Many of these work, at least temporarily, until you stop using them and the body is able to bounce back after being abused. As you may have guessed after understanding your calorie balance system, just because something helps you lose weight does not mean it is good for your health. As I pointed out before, you can lose weight with an advanced case of tuberculosis or even a small cancer. While some weight-reduction measures may be helpful, the harm others can do extends beyond the bad effects of undernutrition. Some have serious adverse effects on a person's health.

The Drug Scene

You need to know that *there is no such thing as a safe pill to help you lose weight*. The first pills used to promote weight loss were related to the actions of epinephrine and stress, and in transmitting impulses from one nerve fiber to the next in the sympathetic nervous system. These naturally-occurring chemicals in your body do increase metabolism. The side effects were not always desirable. Drugs were developed that had an indirect effect on the release of these chemicals. They are the amphetamine drugs, such as Dexedrine (dextro-amphetamine) and Benzedrine (amphetamine sulfate). These are the drugs peo-

221

ple use as "uppers," involved in so much drug abuse. They also suppress your appetite. Technically, these drugs are all modifications of phenethylamine. Because of the undesirable effects of amphetamines, new modifications were synthesized to have less of a stimulant effect, and more of an appetite-suppressing effect. This gave rise to Tenuate and other similar medicines. Unfortunately, most of these modifications still have some effect in stimulating the nervous system. Most can cause a rise in blood pressure, increase in heart rate and even cause significant cardiac irregularities. That is why these medicines should not be used by anyone who has high blood pressure or heart disease.

These drugs suppress the appetite by reacting with receptors in the brain. One of them, fenluramine (Pondimin) is thought to stimulate the release of serotonin in the brain. As I mentioned earlier, serotonin is a chemical called a neurotransmitter. It is present in the hypothalamus where your appetite is controlled. When your serotonin level rises your appetite is suppressed. Although it is a member of the group of drugs that stimulate the sympathetic nervous system, it does not have as much effect on exciting the nervous system as the adrenaline-type preparations. Large doses, though, will cause the same effects as amphetamine. Prolonged use may also cause physical dependence. If a person has been taking this drug for a long time, it should not be stopped abruptly, as that may cause a severe depression.

One of the more popular ingredients in diet pills is phenylpropanolamine. Two popular weight control preparations that contain this drug are Dexatrim and Acutrim. It is also found in a number of medicines for colds, which you can get without a prescription. Some of the appetite suppressing medicines that contain this drug are Dexatrim, Dieutrim, Prolamine and Control. This medicine has been implicated as a possible cause for increased strokes in young people using such pills. One problem may be the individual use of excessive amounts. It has been reported that this drug has caused a number of people to seek help in emergency rooms. The reactions include high blood pressure, anxiety and psychotic episodes. As if having strokes were not bad enough, it also can cause personality changes; there are horror stories such as the one about the person who stripped naked at the airport and other episodes of bizarre behavior.

Caffeine also needs to be mentioned. It is not the same drug, but it is a mild central nervous system stimulant, and is included in the group of medicines called analeptics. In small amounts, it will increase metabolism about 10 percent. It is not entirely without its side effects, either, despite its widespread use.

The diet drugs are helpful in suppressing appetite without sapping a person of energy, which does result in weight loss. Again, it is worth mentioning that losing the weight, in many cases, is not necessarily good. The other question is about how long the weight loss lasts. Once the drugging of the body is stopped, it has the opportunity to re-establish your proper fat level. There is no evidence that any of these diet aids will have any lasting benefit, without taking them indefinitely, which is not safe.

Smoking Off Pounds

It is common knowledge that many people gain weight when they quit smoking. That seems to be particularly true of lean smokers. It is less well-known that about a third of former smokers lose weight, and another third have no change in weight at all. Considering the wide variations of adaptations that can be made to control a person's weight, this inconsistent response should not be too surprising. Nicotine from tobacco does stimulate the release of norepinephrine from nerve endings, the same thing that drugs such as the amphetamine group do. This may also explain the addictive nature of cigarette smoking. For some people, stopping smoking is a lot like getting off speed.

This action of nicotine may have an appetite-suppressive effect. In addition, at least in some people, it has a short-term effect in increasing metabolism, as measured by oxygen consumption. A recent study in Switzerland of individuals who smoked 24 cigarettes in a day showed the increase in energy expenditure. The subjects were all studies inside a metabolic chamber. On the day they smoked, they used an average of 215 calories more than on the days they did not smoke. Since this was not a long-term study, no conclusions can be drawn on what effects would be observed in individuals smoking daily for long periods of time. However, in view of the large number of people who are overweight and do smoke, it seems evident that cigarette smoking is not effective in preventing the accumulation of body fat. There are probably marked individual differences.

In any case, the increased calorie loss, even for the one-day observation, is easily equaled by simply walking three or four miles a day.

That is a great deal healthier than smoking. Even if it were true, which I doubt, that cigarette smoking enabled a person to eliminate over 200 calories a day on a continuous basis, deciding to smoke would be a bad decision. Any benefits that might be gained from controlling body weight by smoking would be greatly outweighed by its bad effects, including chronic lung disease, cancer of the lungs and a three-fold increase in the risk of having a heart attack or a stroke. Clearly cigarettes are not a good medicine to use to lose weight.

If you smoke, and decide to quit, you can help insure yourself against gaining weight by simply decreasing your calorie intake a small amount and increasing your exercise a little bit. For most people, all three measures—quitting smoking, decreasing calorie intake and increasing physical activity—are steps along the right road to good health. For those thin people who gain weight when they quit smoking, one must guess that they have recovered from the toxic effects of tobacco and have regained their proper weight. In others, the need to do something results in serious overeating, which is temporary and needs to be controlled.

Stay Up All Night and Lose Weight

We use more calories during the day than we do at night. That is related to the diurnal cycle and the hours of sleep. The body temperature is lowest during the early morning hours of sleep, when the body uses the least energy. The metabolic fires are banked during the night. As the day progresses, the temperature rises, as does energy use, until the temperature hits its peak in the late afternoon or early evening. If you change your hours of sleep and activity, the temperature cycle and energy cycle also change. Studies show that you will use 10 to 13 percent less energy when you are asleep than you use when you are awake but in the near-basal state. If you stay up all night, you will never reach the basal state, and will continue to use additional calories. That, of course, is neither possible nor desirable on a long-term basis. But it does point out that the fewer hours a person sleeps, the more calories he will use on a daily basis.

A person who is eating normally will have more energy, and be more likely to stay up and be involved in a number of activities. That, in turn, enables him to use more calories. In a way, if you have energy, you will use energy. You can also see why people who stay up late at

night, particularly doing something besides watching TV, may begin
to lose weight. This is often noted in young people who are out every
night, as long as being out doesn't also include taking on extra calories.

The Horrible Hormones

One of the methods to lose body fat that has been touted as a miracle
is human chorionic gonadotropin, otherwise known as HCG. This is a
hormone secreted by the structures surrounding the implanted, fertil-
ized ovum. It resembles the action of one of the pituitary hormones
(luteinizing hormone). A popular approach to treating overweight was
to give injections of HCG and impose a 500-calorie diet. It was reported that this program caused a weight loss of 9 to 14 kilograms (20
to 31 pounds) in 40 days. When you consider the water loss, protein
loss and emptying of the intestines, that might be possible in a person
who required 2,700 calories a day. But the weight loss is not related to
the HCG. A number of studies of the effects of HCG have shown that
it is no more effective than a placebo—a nonmedical inert preparation
with no action.

The other hormone touted to help people lose weight is growth hormone. Growth hormone is normally produced by the pituitary gland.
Certainly, growth uses calories. When growth hormone has been given
to children who have decreased pituitary function, it does result in loss
of subcutaneous fat and stimulates growth. It will also increase metabolism. Until recently, human growth hormone was simply not available, except for severe problems in growth. More recently, growth hormone has been synthesized, and its effects can be studied in greater
depth. But there is a problem, as mentioned before. Since growth hormone stimulates growth, and an adult's bones have calcified so that
linear growth can't occur, the hormone will cause acromegaly, a condition of enlargement of the hands, feet and face bones. This endocrine
disease causes other medical disorders.

Growth hormone is one of the newest hormone preparations to be
sold on the black market. It is a complex substance that is normally
produced by the body. The brain forms a growth hormone releasing
hormone (GHRH) which allows your pituitary to release growth hormone. Then the growth hormone acts on substances in your liver to
produce still another substance that actually stimulates growth. It used

to be thought that growth hormone was produced only during your growth years, but we now know that it is still produced after growth stops. Exactly what it does after growth is not clear. But the "body people" claim it will melt fat away and grow muscles. The catch is that if you start taking growth hormone, it will decrease the normal amount produced by your pituitary, just as taking thyroid hormone decreases the thyroid gland's function in a normal person. If you did take enough growth hormone to exceed your normal production, you would not like the results. In young people it can stimulate the growth of giants and produce deformities. In the mature adult it causes changes I have mentioned called acromegaly.

Fortunately, the products that have been available on the black market are so weak they have no significant effect. The preparation has to be kept refrigerated to be active. Some preparations sold as growth hormone actually are just distilled water. There may be a place for the further study of the effects of growth hormone on muscle development. It is likely that strength training uses up the muscle stores of certain chemicals and that in turn stimulates the action of growth hormone to activate substances that stimulate muscle growth. But these concepts are in the research phase and there is no place for the use of growth hormone obtained on the black market.

Related to growth hormone is the amino acid scene. The two amino acids of greatest interest are arginine and ornithine. In large amounts they are thought to stimulate the release of growth hormone, which in turn causes you to shed pounds of fat and develop pounds of bulging muscles. It's a real sales pitch that appeals to those interested in "burning off fat" and growing muscles, as this letter shows.

> DEAR DR. LAMB: I am an 18-year-old male in good health except for being 25 to 30 pounds overweight. I've been trying to lose this excess fat for about two years. I've been active in athletics and have been involved with an exercise program where I run two to three miles five days a week. Also, I work out with weights three days a week.
>
> I cut out almost all fatty foods, sugars, sweets, fried foods and high calorie foods. I've done this for almost two years and haven't lost a pound of fat. I have gained some muscle. Why is this and how can I permanently shed this excess fat? Are fat burning products using amino acids any good? I'm stumped.

The amino acid pitch appeals to young men wanting to "muscle-up" also because many have been sold on taking protein supplements as an aid to growing muscles—which they don't need either if they plan their diet properly.

The amino acid products that people can buy are taken by mouth. Here is one of the traps that often occur about substances people consume that are supposed to have magic results. It makes a lot of difference whether something is injected or swallowed. Anything that is swallowed must first pass through your digestive system and then be absorbed into your circulation before it has any effect. When the substance is digested or incompletely absorbed, it doesn't have the same effect as when taken by injection. That is true of swallowing amino acids. The preparations that are currently being sold for high prices contain such small amounts compared to what would be required for oral administration that they are unlikely to have any significant effect. I do not recommend taking these products.

I have already told you about using thyroid hormone in the hopes of losing weight. Thyroid hormone replacement is important in people who have a hypothyroid condition, whether they are overweight or not. Otherwise, taking thyroid to lose weight is either useless or downright dangerous, depending on how much you take and other factors.

Intestinal Bypass

It's hard to believe this operation was ever done. Yet, it is still used in treating the morbidly obese, who have a high risk of severe medical problems or death unless drastic measures are taken. It is usually not considered unless a person is at least 110 pounds overweight, and conservative measures to control gross obesity have failed.

Regardless of which operative procedure is used, the purpose is to let the food bypass a major portion of the small intestine. In essence, the operation creates a situation where absorption of the food that enters the intestine is decreased. That is why patients who have had this operation usually have many of the features of a malabsorption disease, such as sprue or pancreatic failure with diarrhea. It seems clear that if you consume calories, but they are never absorbed, you might as well not have consumed them at all, as far as your energy balance system is concerned.

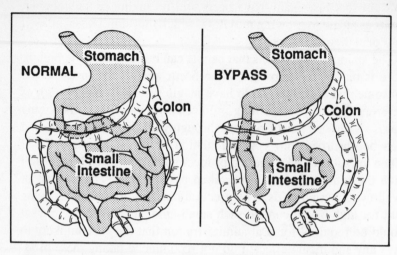

The intestinal bypass operation converts much of the small intestine into a blind segment of bowel which the food to be digested does not enter.

Since most digestion occurs in the very first segment of the small intestine, just outside the stomach, the effects of an intestinal bypass are not as marked as you might expect, even though a major portion of the small intestine is bypassed. Studies show that the operation prevents the absorption of about 450 calories a day. This is equivalent to the calories in only about 58 grams of body fat a day, or 21 kilograms (46 pounds) in a year. A 154-pound (70 kilogram) person would use the calories in a little more than 50 pounds, in the same year's time, if he walked 8 miles a day. Since the people considered for an intestinal bypass are grossly obese, and weigh more, they would not need to walk nearly as great a distance. Unfortunately, many of the people who are candidates for this operation are not medically able to perform that much activity.

Intestinal bypass patients often lose much more weight. Some lose over 100 kilograms (220 pounds). The amount of weight loss is affected by the length of intestine bypassed, and other factors. The weight loss over and above that accounted for by plain failure to absorb nutrients is mostly from a decreased food intake. You might think that because of the decreased absorption that the appetite would increase enough to offset the loss, but that does not happen. The weight loss that occurs is usually permanent. In successful cases, life-threatenting situations such as very high blood pressure and cholesterol are improved.

The drawbacks to this form of surgery are many, and that is why it is not used unless necessary. The interpretation of "necessary" is subject to debate. There are other ways to reduce even the morbidly obese person with serious medical complications. It is expected that all bypass patients will have severe postoperative diarrhea of as many as 20 stools a day. This gradually subsides to only two to six stools a day within six months. Medicines to control the diarrhea are needed.

The malabsorption, like that seen in medical diseases, results in vitamin and mineral deficiencies, particularly vitamin B-12 and the fat-soluble vitamins A and E. There may be a decrease in blood proteins because of inadequate absorption of amino acids from protein foods.

The list doesn't end there. Some patients develop serious liver disease. Others have a bacterial overgrowth in their intestines, causing a serious clinical situation, and some develop a form of arthritis.

It's pretty evident that intestinal bypass surgery is not going to be the solution for most people's problem of being overweight.

Shrinking the Stomach

There are several surgical procedures designed to decrease the capacity of the stomach. These have some merit, because when the stomach is distended, stretch fibers of the nervous system relay a signal to the brain to shut down the appetite. However, none of these procedures should be considered, except in people who are grossly obese and have been unsuccessful in reversing the condition with conservative management. I do receive a number of letters asking about these procedures, like this one from the lady who writes,

DEAR DR. LAMB: Are you familiar with a surgical procedure called gastric segmentation, used for the treatment of obesity? If yes, what is your opinion of the procedure? Is it safe? Is it successful?

I have had gastric stapling done for obesity and it was not successful. I am 150 pounds overweight, a compulsive eater, and 55 years old. What is your advice? And please don't tell me to go on a sensible diet and get rid of the excess weight. You have been a physician long enough to know there is no long-range success in that advice.

Notice that she has had gastric stapling and it was not successful. That was the early stage in the development of this procedure. Although it received a lot of publicity regarding how successful it was—it wasn't. The first simple operation was to just staple across the top of the stomach, leaving a space that was not stapled as a hole, to allow food to pass from the chamber above the line of staples into the lower chamber. A major problem was that the staples often opened. That occurred as early as the first week after the operation. The staples opened in 67 to 81 percent of the patients and that allowed them to return to their previous level of food intake, and the operation was a failure.

The next attempt was to prevent the opening of the staples by suturing them in place. That resulted in frequent problems of vomiting and dehydration. Many patients had to be hospitalized and the opening dialated. The size of the opening proved critical. If it was less than 1.0 cm the patients couldn't tolerate even semisolid food, but if it was larger than 1.5 cm the patients could eat normal amounts of food. Also the opening would sometimes undergo progressive scarring, causing obstruction.

Then came the third adaptation, making a vertical partition. This did decrease the vomiting but 11 percent of patients still had to have the opening dialated.

There is still another option, which is a gastric bypass. The top of the stomach is completely closed off leaving it as a separate pouch. A segment of the first end of the small intestine is attached to the upper small pouch. That means food would accumulate in the small stomach pouch, then pass through the small intestine, bypassing the lower large stomach chamber. The outlet of the lower chamber is also attached to the small intestine so its contents can drain normally into the intestine. It has been reported that the morbidly obese, those between 202 and 505 pounds, have lost more than 100 pounds in some cases. The vertical partition procedure is said to cause a loss of 27 percent of the body weight.

A person having a vertical partition or the stomach bypass procedure should expect some complications. Doctors have been familiar for years with the effects of mechanically shrinking the stomach. It has long been a standard procedure to surgically remove a major

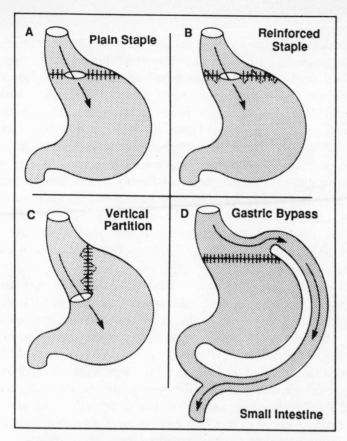

A. The simple stapling operation. **B.** Staples reinforced with sutures. **C.** The vertical stapling procedure. **D.** The gastric pouch or segmentation method of decreasing effective stomach capacity.

portion of the stomach in some patients with severe peptic ulcer problems that cannot be managed medically. This is a partial gastrectomy. A common complication after the operation is the "dumping syndrome." This results in flushing, a rapid heart beat, faintness and diarrhea. I would recommend that anyone considering any of these procedures think hard about alternative, less traumatic methods of losing weight.

Ballooning the Stomach

There is still another way you can shut off your appetite by stimulating the stretch fibers in the stomach, without having surgery or stapling your stomach. You can have a balloon put inside your stomach. The idea was first tried by Drs. Ole G. Niebin and Henrik Harboe of Denmark. They placed a balloon inside the stomach, then inflated it to a volume of about one pint. They said they got the idea from the effects of bezoars. These are undigested materials that lodge in the stomach and form a solid mass, like a soft stone. At one time, they were thought to have magical healing powers—outside the stomach not inside it. Queen Elizabeth I of England had several for their medicinal powers. Inside the stomach, they can cause symptoms of obstruction. But, more often, they simply cause weight loss. Indeed, with a 10-day trial of the gastric balloon Drs. Niebin and Harboe's subjects lost as much as 11 pounds.

Since the original work, others have tried the same or a similar procedure of putting an inflated balloon inside the stomach. It has been used for as long as four months, then deflated and removed. Of course, the patients have to go on a diet, too. It is the diet, or the decreased calorie intake, that causes the weight loss. You could have the same effect without the balloon if you were willing to stay on the same low-calorie diet. The one advantage of the balloon is that it provides that full feeling from stomach distention before you eat so much. It just makes it easier to stay on a low calorie diet. Again, there is no magic, just a limitation of calorie intake.

You might think this is a wonderful idea, but after the initial enthusiasm the problems began to appear. It caused perforations and ulcers of the stomach, intestinal blockages and even one reported death. If it deflates after it is in the stomach it must be removed and that may require surgery. If it is not removed immediately the results may be fatal. About 2 percent of one balloon, known as a gastric bubble, deflated with three months. These complications led the manufacturer to recommend to physicians not to use the bubble except in extreme cases where other measures had failed.

Suck It Out, Cut It Off

I have already mentioned that if you don't like those rolls of fat around your trunk, or over your buttocks and thighs, you can take the direct approach and just have the fat cut off. It's called body sculpturing, and it is not without merit. Of course, it is done as a cosmetic procedure, but let's face it, the main reason many people want to get rid of fat is to look better. This is not a simple procedure, as handling the skin and the fat deposits requires skill and experience. Remember that the skin is extremely vascular. There are a lot of nerves and blood vessels that pass through the body fat to the skin. That is how it functions as the heat-exchanger to eliminate calories from your body. There is always the danger of shock from the removal of the fat. Body sculpturing may leave long scars, as it is necessary for the surgeon to see what he is doing. At the same time he can remove excess skin, to avoid the problem of sagging, unsightly folds of skin that often follows losing lots of fat.

Liposuction was originally developed in Paris and it was done with a long, blunt stiff probe. It has been used in the United States now for over five years. During that time, many refinements in the technique have been accomplished. One of the most important has been the development of small flexible probes. These allow the doctor to remove small amounts of fat from critical areas. They are particularly useful in removing fat from the face, literally allowing the surgeon to sculpt a new look.

Liposuction is a blind procedure, and consists of making a small incision in the skin and inserting the probe. The probe is hollow, and is a suction device. With suction, the soft fat is sucked into the device and eliminated. This procedure appeals to many because of the small scar that it makes. The early large probe made tunnels in the layers of fat and could leave the body with a rippled effect like your grandmother's washboard. There is still the problem of excess skin. You can't get rid of excess skin without cutting it off. If you have excess skin to start with, removing underlying fat will just make the appearance worse. Liposuction is not used for generalized large fat deposits. In a recent review of the five years' experience with liposuction, The American Society of Plastic and Reconstructive Surgeons pointed out that removing as little as 1,500 ml of fat tissue (about three pounds) could result in shock from fluid shifts. They recommended that no more than 2,000 ml of fat be removed at one time on an outpatient basis. Removing this amount or more needs to be done under a general anesthetic in the hospital prepared to deal with such complications as shock. You have to wait six months before it is safe to have it done again. At that rate, it will take a long time to remove 100 pounds of excess body fat by liposuction. Its best use is the remove the small rolls of fat that persist after a weight control program and seem to be the most reluctant to melt away.

The review of complications connected with liposuction revealed that in 100,000 cases there were 11 deaths. Deaths can occur from infections and blood clots or fat emboli that travel through the heart and to the lungs, causing a pulmonary embolism and shock.

It is important to remember that about half of the body fat is inside the body, not under the skin. Regardless of how much fat you remove with either body sculpturing or liposuction, the fat inside the body will be unaffected.

You might ask if the fat will come back. Keep in mind that the adult already has all the fat cells he is going to have. Remember Hirsch and colleagues' experiments at Rockefeller University. They showed that if you removed half of the fat deposits from part of a litter of rats, they did not get fat like their unoperated littermates when they both ate the same diet. Considering the concept that fat cells have different receptors that control whether or not they will give up their fat deposits easily, there is a good possibility that one way of eliminating the tendency to fat deposits under the skin would be just to remove the cells. If Hirsch is right, and there is a feed-back mechanism between fat cells and the brain, this would also stop the stimulation from fat cells that drives the appetite until those cells are filled with the desired amount of fat.

Wrapping It Up

One of the more ill-advised approaches to losing body fat is to use wrappers or even to use plastic sweat suits. I receive many letters asking about the benefits of these. One person wrote,

> DEAR DR. LAMB: I saw an item in a Believe It Or Not that caught my eye. It claimed that actor Don McLeod wore a gorilla suit that weighed 35 pounds and he lost seven pounds a day when he wore it. How could that be? If it is true, where can I get a cheaper gorilla suit? I note his cost $20,000.00.
>
> I would certainly like to lose seven pounds a day. Since I don't have $20,000.00 for a gorilla suit, could you send me a diet program to help

me lose about 20 pounds? I don't expect to lose seven pounds a day, so I
want to get started now to be ready for summer when it gets here.

Although Don McLeod may have lost seven pounds in one day,
you know from what you have learned that it was not fat. It was
water. And that means after the day was over and he replenished his
body's water needs, he gained back a lot or all of the weight before
the next time he had to wear the gorilla suit. The suit no doubt
worked like many sweat garments people wear in the hopes of losing weight. These do not help you lose a single pound of fat.

As you now know, the body eliminates calories through your
skin. When you wrap up the skin all you do is make it more difficult
for your air conditioner to work. Think again about my original
analogy of a room air condition stuck through the wall. If you went
outside and wrapped it, it couldn't blow hot air out and cool the
room. If you wrap up your skin, it will have trouble giving up heat
too. Such garments can actually be dangerous. If the body cannot
eliminate heat properly, your body temperature will rise, and if it
rises high enough you can have a heat stroke.

Then there are the local wraps that have been promoted, which
this lady writes about.

> DEAR DR. LAMB: I am a tall woman, 5 feet 11, and weigh 253
> pounds, which is too much even for my height. For the past five months
> I have been on a 1,300 calorie diet and exercise faithfully, but have lost
> only about six pounds.
>
> My weight is mainly in the middle, stomach, hips and thighs. I have
> no health problems and am in my mid-50s. Recently a friend recom-
> mended "body wrapping" to eliminate cellulite. Is this a good thing
> healthwise, or would you recommend staying with a good food and
> exercise program?

Such local wraps have only a local effect and it is not on fat loss.
You can induce localized sweating of the skin. You can eliminate
some local water under the skin. That is why bodybuilders use such
devices just before competition, to eliminate local normal water and
cause a better definition of the muscles. Applying heat does not
cause a loss of body heat. The truth is just the opposite. When you
expose yourself to cold and lose more calories through the skin, you
lose weight or must increase your calorie intake. I cannot recom-

mend body wrapping for anything more than whatever pleasure a person gets from it, just as they do with various means of heat application, including lying in the sun.

People often come to the wrong conclusions about what helps them lose weight. There is a tendency to think that some special thing they did was the real secret. That is how a lot of misconceptions get started. This is a typical misconception.

> DEAR DR. LAMB: I am 25 years old, 5 feet 10 inches tall and weigh 187 pounds. I have lost 85 pounds in the last two years and I did it all the wrong way. I mean I stopped eating pork, eggs and cut down on the sweets, but my exercise was handled wrong. I started walking and then running wearing a plastic bag and I still do it.
>
> What I need to know is what is my ideal weight for my height and age? Can I maintain such weight by just leaving sugar and bread completely alone and not using the bag to sweat?

This young man did not lose fat because of the plastic bag. Stop and consider what he has told us. He lost 85 pounds in 104 weeks, far less than one pound a week. And he cut down or eliminated the high-calorie foods in his diet as well as followed an exercise program. A combination of decreased calorie consumption and increased calorie expenditure through exercise can very easily cause a motivated person to lose that much weight a week. What he needs to do is stay on a sensible diet and exercise program. If he needs to lose still more body fat, he should concentrate on building up both his endurance and strength exercise program to help him. He needs to build up his metabolic furnace so he can eat normally without being overweight.

Summary 17

1. There is no such thing as a safe, effective pill to cause you to lose body fat.
2. Most pills taken to cause a loss of weight contain substances that are related to amphetamines, "uppers," and may cause high blood pressure. Some cause anxiety and even bizarre behavior.
3. Smoking cigarettes does help some people avoid being overweight, but the cost in terms of lung disease, cancer, and a three-

fold increase in the risk of heart attacks and strokes greatly out-
weighs the benefits.

4. You use fewer calories when you are asleep than when you are
   awake, and lack of sleep can cause weight loss, unless a person
   consumes more calories while still awake.
5. All of the hormone preparations suggested for losing weight are
   either ineffective or dangerous in larger amounts.
6. Amino acid preparations available to the public at great expense
   are ineffective and do not "burn off fat while you sleep."
7. The intestinal bypass operation to eliminate gross obesity is effective, but also causes many very serious side effects.
8. Surgery on the stomach to decrease its storage capacity has a
   checkered history and has been both useless and harmful. However, some of the newer methods are helpful in treating the morbidly obese who cannot otherwise eliminate excess body fat.
9. Putting a balloon in the stomach seemed like a good idea, but
   dangerous complications resulting from this have made it a very
   questionable procedure.
10. Liposuction and other surgical procedures to remove excess body
    fat are an option in selected cases, especially for people with small
    areas of fat that are resistant to weight control measures.
11. Body wraps and plastic bags do not eliminate body fat, only the
    body's normal water content, and they can be dangerous.

Chapter 18

When You Want to Gain Weight

DEAR DR. LAMB: I have read many letters in your column from people wanting to lose weight. The whole world seems to be obsessed with losing weight. There are ads about how to lose weight and books about how to lose weight. But how in the world do you gain weight?

I am a real broomstick. I'm 35 years old, 5 feet 4 inches tall and only weigh 96 pounds. All my life I have been skinny. I don't have any shape. Dresses don't fit because they don't make clothes for people like me. I'm not talking about having big breasts. I'm talking about not having any fat anywhere. Some women complain because their behind is too big. Let me tell those women something, it is better to have a big behind than not to have any at all. I'm flat. So flat that it hurts to sit on a hard chair.

I've tried to eat a lot and I think I have a good well-balanced diet. Even when I force myself to eat, I don't gain weight. Yes, I've been to the doctor, not one doctor but several, and they all say I'm in perfect health. I have lots of energy and am very active. My only problem is I can't gain weight. Do you have any suggestions?

Although the major preoccupation today is with losing weight, there are a few people who have exactly the opposite problem. They want to gain weight. In many instances, they have trouble gaining weight for exactly the same reason other people have for losing weight. They have a built-in range for a body weight that is normal for them, and their energy balance system adjusts itself to keep them within that range—which is on the thin side. Most of the people who write me about wanting to gain weight are young males

239

who feel they need to "beef up," or are concerned about their relatively thin stature. When a young girl worries about this, it is usually because she has not developed normal fat pads, and does not have the figure she thinks she should have. Some continue to be thin, at least until the menopause, and are distressed with their thin state—as the woman in the letter is—the entire time. In some cases, it is a particular feature they are distressed about, such as having thin legs that "look like toothpicks." This woman evidently failed to develop normal fat distribution, which she should have done when she entered puberty. It is worth evaluating her hormone balance. There are important quesitons, such as whether she has regular menstrual periods or not and whether she has had children, which would provide answers as to how normally her hormone system has developed. If she has normal menstrual cycles, it is unlikely that an estrogen deficiency is the problem. It is more likely that she has inherited the genes to be thin and will be until her life script for body weight dictates that she can weigh more.

There is still another aspect of being thin—unintentional weight loss. This often means there is a significant medical problem, or it may follow surgery. The patient realizes that he or she is too thin and needs to regain weight. Regardless of the cause, the principles involved in gaining weight are the same as those used to lose weight.

If you want to gain weight, you must decide what kind of weight you want to gain. You could resort to being inactive and eat, eat, eat. That will usually lead to weight gain. The weight gain will be fat. You need to ask yourself if you really want to add pounds of fat to your body. What will it look like under your skin? Are you concerned about the effect extra fat might have upon your total cholesterol, blood pressure and other aspects of your health? Do you want to be a human version of the feed-lot animal? If you have completed your normal growth cycle, you are not groing to grow any taller, just rounder.

If you don't want to add pounds of fat to your body, the other choice is to grow muscles. That is the healthy way to gain weight. It requires strength training, and that is true for both males and females. Males respond better to strength training in terms of developing muscles simply because men produce more testosterone and testosterone stimulates muscle development.

Unintentional Weight Loss

Anyone who has unexplained weight loss needs a complete medical evaluation. It starts with a diet diary, which lists all the sources of calories a person consumes. Sometimes, unexplained weight loss happens because a person actually is not getting enough calories. This is particularly apt to occur in a person who lives alone, or in an older individual who has lost the zest for eating. When the calorie intake is too low, it is important to examine why. In some instances it is because of depression. When a person gets depressed, he or she frequently has a loss of appetite. Often, a depressed person doesn't consume enough calories, and loses weight. The gaunt face of weight loss accentuates the appearance of depression.

It is equally important to have an activity diary, to estimate how many calories a person is using a day. In a young person, it may be that constant activity without an adequate calorie intake can result in being thin. A strength-training program to build muscles will not be successful if you jog, run, play sports, and are so active that it is difficult to have a calorie intake large enough to support your daily needs. The young woman who says she has been thin all her life needs to examine both whether she really consumes enough calories and how many calories she is using with her activity. Her statement that she is very active could mean she is using a lot of calories.

The medical evaluation must include a search for serious illness. In a recent study by Dr. Mordechai Rabinovitz and colleagues from Tel Aviv University in Israel, the cause of unintentional weight loss in 154 patients was analyzed. The most frequent cause was cancer—56 percent.

Almost half of these cancers were of the digestive system. The next largest group, 26 percent, was of patients with a variety of diseases of the digestive tract, other than cancer. Almost half of these were ulcers. Another 16 percent had psychiatric disorders, and more than a third of these were patients with a depression. Another 20 percent had a variety of disorders, including infectious disease, hyperthyroidism (less than 2 percent) and diabetes (less than 2 percent). Even after a searching medical examination, the cause of weight loss was unexplained in 36 percent. This survey points out some important features of unintentional weight loss. It usually means a person has a medical problem that needs attention. And unintentional weight loss does occur even when the cause is not explained. It is also interesting to note that hyperthyroidism and diabetes were not common causes for unexplained weight loss. Of course both should be considered in anyone who has a history of unexplained weight loss. More often these people will have been of normal weight and then have a weight loss, rather than having failed to gain weight in the first place. The frequency of cancer as the reason for unintentional weight loss emphasizes the importance of a person with this problem having a searching medical examination.

The role of depression deserves some emphasis as a cause for weight loss, even though it was not a frequent cause in the Israeli series. Depression is a common condition, particularly in middle-aged and older people. It can be quite serious and should not be overlooked. It does not have to cause a person to look severely depressed, or to be sitting in the corner crying constantly. It can occur in a person and not be recognized by those around him. It is often denied even by the person who is depressed. Don't be too quick to dismiss it as a possible cause for a person's loss of appetite. As more has been learned about brain chemistry, it is clear that a decrease of important chemicals within the brain can be a major cause of depression. The two chemicals of prime importance are serotonin and norepinephrine. These are called monamines. As their level is restored within the brain, the depression lifts. When that happens, the person's appetite returns. The antidepressant medicines used to treat these conditions increase the level of these monamines in the brain. They may also cause a significant weight gain.

Eating to Gain Weight

If you have lost a lot of muscle from an illness, or for whatever reason, you will want to include enough protein in your diet to help support muscle growth. As I suggested, for muscle development at a rate of one pound a week, that means you need about 100 grams (3-1/2 ounces) of good quality protein a day. See chapter 13, Putting Muscle Into Your Calorie Balance, for more information. You will also need enough calories so that the protein in your diet can be used for growth, rather than being used to meet calorie needs.

It is muscle that most men want to develop, certainly not fat. It is not just the young man who wants muscles. Older men hate to see their muscular shape change and disappear. In a sense it is equated to a loss of manhood. A major reason for the loss of muscles as people get older is failure to use their muscles in a way that requires strength. This man expresses the common feeling that many men have.

DEAR DR. LAMB: I'm a male, 79 years old and in good health. My blood pressure is 112/80, my heart is good and all my vital signs are good. I'm 5 feet 11 inches tall and weigh only 135 pounds. I would like to gain about 20 pounds, but have not been able to. My weight has not fluctuated more than five pounds in the last 20 years. I understand the thyroid gland has something to do with this. Is there any way to activate this condition. I have not smoked for over 20 years.

Since this man's weight has not fluctuated more than five pounds in 20 years we know that he was this thin at age 59 and possibly much before that. That pretty well rules out any serious medical cause for his low body weight, such as cancer or even diabetes. It is unlikely that he would have had an overactive thyroid all that time without it being recognized, but of course that is one of the things that should be looked for. He probably inherited the genes to weigh this amount at his age. A doctor friend once reminded me years ago that when he went to Florida and saw lots of older people, he noticed that very few of them were overweight. That is certainly consistent with the studies that have been done on body weight and longevity. So this man should be happy that he is on the lean side and has had a stable weight all these years. He might be able to slowly increase his muscle size with a carefully planned exercise program.

To add fat to your body, you need more calories than your body uses. It doesn't matter if you inherited a tendency to be thin, you can override your characteristics if you really want to do so. The trick is to consume calorie-rich foods. The situation is a lot like the regular laboratory rats that had no inherited tendency to get fat. As long as they ate their regular mixed diet, they didn't get enough calories to get fat, but when that diet was substituted or supplemented with food rich in calories, they got fat. The rats that were designed genetically to be fat got fat on either diet.

To add pounds of fat, you need to eat the very foods that you should avoid to keep from getting fat. The number one food in that category is fat itself. It contains more calories per gram than anything else you can eat. It is already packaged in such a way that when it is not used for daily energy requirements, it can be immediately processed and stored in your fat cells. It is far better, in terms of trying to gain body fat, than starches, sweets or concentrated carbohydrates. If you consume too much extra carbohydrate, it is more likely to drive your energy system and release more calories that must be eliminated through your skin. Remember that carbohydrates prevent the slowdown in thyroid function that people experience when they are on a calorie-restricted diet. The slowdown occurs on those low-carbohydrate diets composed of fat and protein. Nevertheless, those starches, sweets and concentrated carbohydrate foods, in excess of your calorie needs, do contribute to gaining body fat.

You want to avoid the low-calorie foods that will fill your stomach and curtail your appetite. Salads are great foods for health, but not so great for gaining weight, unless they are laced with a high-calorie salad dressing.

What about vitamins and minerals to help you gain weight? Forget it. You need the proper amount of these for good nutrition, but none of these will help you gain extra body fat or develop new muscles. For the most part, the role of vitamins is similar to that of the spark plug in an engine. The spark is essential to burn the fuel, but it is not the source of the energy. Vitamins are the spark to stimulate the burning of your hydrocarbon fuel, but they are not the source of energy. If the spark plugs are bad, an engine will not use gasoline efficiently, and it will be low on energy. Likewise, if you do not have the proper level of the right vitamins, you will not be able to burn your hydrocarbon fuel properly, and you will be low on energy. But never be misled into thinking the vitamins are the source of the energy.

There is little else you can do with your diet to force your body to gain weight, and I have to ask again, are you sure you really want to do this?

Physical Activity and Weight Gain

Exercise can be a great aid in either gaining or losing weight. It depends on how you use it, and your goal. If you like to jog or run, you are not likely to gain weight if you do a lot of it. These endurance exercises are calorie burners. They stimulate your body to eliminate calories, not to retain them to build muscle. It follows that if a person really is too thin, these exercises should be used only in moderation, or not at all. The laborer who must be active all day will lose weight unless he consumes an enormous number of calories. The number he needs will be directly related to the number of calories his body uses.

The way to develop muscles is to follow a good strength-training program. It must be followed without using all your calorie intake for endurance exercises. There is a right and a wrong way to do these exercises, and to be successful. See chapter 13, Putting Muscle into Your Calorie Balance, for more information on developing muscles. Once you have developed your muscle size, you must maintain a proper exercise routine to keep them. They will also enable you to eat a high-calorie diet and not gain fat. There is an important distinction between gaining body fat and gaining muscle size. The increased muscle size is usually healthy, but the increased body fat stores may not be.

Habits Are Important

Certain habits can be a factor in causing a person to be thin. High on the list is cigarette smoking. If a person wants to gain weight, and is thin, it is important to stop smoking. Everyone should stop anyway, for other reasons. It is the skinny cigarette smoker who has the highest risk of death before his time, and he is is also the one who is apt to gain weight when he stops smoking. Remember that nicotine may have an appetite-suppression action and may stimulate metabolism slightly. It is also a cellular poison. That is another reason why a person who smokes may be thin—he is literally poisoning his body cells. For the person who already has a normal body weight, or is overweight, stopping smoking may not cause an increase in body weight.

Coffee, tea and caffeine-containing colas may detract from a person's ability to gain weight. Caffeine enhances the action of epinephrine and may also have a mild appetite-suppressant action. It may increase the metabolism slightly, and in this way contribute to the release of calories.

Remember that your metabolism is at low ebb when you are asleep. Since the goal in gaining weight is to be in positive calorie balance, you want to take advantage of situations that will enhance this. If you need to gain weight, be sure to get a proper amount of sleep regularly.

You have seen that cold will cause the body to lose more calories and stimulate metabolism. It is not surprising that a person who is thin and wants to be either comfortable, or to gain weight, should dress warmly when exposed to the cold. Will you gain weight, then, if you are hot? No. Look at your electric bills for the summer when you are using air conditioning and you will have the answer. It requires energy to cool your body, just the same as it requires energy to heat the body. The amount of energy required to cool the body is not equal to the amount used to maintain body heat. The burden falls mostly on the heart, which must pump an increased amount of blood through the skin for the cooling effect, whereas the heating is accomplished by almost all cells of the body, and especially by the muscles during physical work. But it is true that to set the optimum conditions for gaining weight, you need to keep the body in an environment that is neither too hot nor too cold, and does not pose an energy rip-off to either heat or cool your body.

Hormones and Weight Gain

In a person who has hyperthyroidism, the simplest way to correct being underweight is to slow down the thyroid gland's activity. By decreasing the number of calories of heat generated by the cells, you can tilt the calorie balance back to normal, and the body will recover its normal weight level. But most individuals who want to gain weight, and are having trouble doing it, do not have an overactive thyroid gland. It is similar to the fact mentioned earlier that most people who are overweight do not have hypothyroidism.

A few women are thin because of low hormone levels. This may occur early in life. A girl may not develop the normal fat deposits that she should at the expected time of puberty because of an inadequate production of estrogen. There may be a defect in the brain-pituitary-ovary mechanism. Usually, when this occurs, there will also be some abnormalities in the menstrual cycle, or menstruation may not occur at all. In these cases a medical evaluation of the hormone balance is important. Correcting any problems that exist will usually result in the development of normal fat deposits.

A similar problem may occur after puberty. There is the situation of they young woman who is an active athlete—which may include being a ballet dancer or a marathon runner—who is thin and doesn't menstruate. Undernutrition may be the culprit. It is important for these women to also be evaluated for a possible hormone imbalance. Rarely, a woman will develop this condition insidiously after giving birth. The pituitary gland may have been damaged during labor. As a result, the brain-pituitary-other endocrine glands mechanism may not work properly. It may affect more than just the ovaries. The associated decrease in function of a number of endocrine glands usually signals that something is wrong. Replacing the needed hormones often corrects the situation. Estrogen does not stimulate the growth of muscle and cannot be used to help a woman develop her muscle size. Testosterone can in most cases, but neither testosterone nor the anabolic steroids should be used for this purpose.

Anabolic steroids do have an important place in medicine. Remember that testosterone does stimulate muscle development. That is the basis for males tending to be more muscular than women. It is harder for women to develop muscles. Their muscles are not likely to be as big and strong as those noted in men. That is also why a woman who uses strength training to improve her muscles may not develop large, bulging biceps. She is more apt to have strong, firm, smaller muscles.

The stimulation of anabolic metabolism by testosterone has many uses, though the associated sexual side effects of facial hair, deeper voice and other masculine characteristics are not always wanted. To have the anabolic benefits, and avoid these complications, synthetic hormones have been developed. These are the anabolic steroids. These preparations may be used in debilitated patients who need to regain body tissue. They are also misused by many athletes to try to improve their competitive edge.

Unfortunately, anabolic steroids are not entirely free of the sexual effects of testosterone. They have important side effects that need to be avoided. That includes possible sterility and liver function damage. In the older male, they may stimulate more rapid enlargement of the prostate gland and lead to prostatic enlargement, causing obstruction to the outflow of urine. They may also contribute to problems of cancer of the prostate. Their use to gain weight or strength should be discouraged. On the other hand, the young male who is deficient in testosterone can benefit from adequate testosterone replacement, or measures that stimulate testosterone production.

When All Else Fails

If you are thin, healthy and have a healthy lifestyle with good nutrition, but an adequate intake of calories and strength exercises do not result in a normal weight gain, it is best to face reality. It is like the healthy person who is "overweight" by most standards because he or she inherited genes that called for that body weight normally. You need to accept what you look like and who you are. *Weighing less or more than arbitrary standards is perfectly all right if it is not an indication of a health problem or increases the risk of a health problem.*

Summary 18

1. The principles in gaining weight are the same principles involved in losing weight and the healthy thin person usually inherits the genes to be thin.
2. Unintentional weight loss requires a medical examination because there is frequently a medical cause.
3. A mental depression is often an unrecognized cause for not eating properly and losing weight.
4. Other medical causes include cancer and diseases of the digestive system, particularly peptic ulcers. An overactive thyroid is a relatively infrequent cause, as is diabetes.
5. When you want to regain lost muscle, which may have resulted from an illness or surgery, you need to be sure you have enough protein to support growth. If you want to gain body fat—which may not be desirable—you need to eat high-calorie foods and fat is a good choice. But it is necessary to guard against raising the total cholesterol level and blood pressure.
6. The healthy way to gain weight is to increase your muscle size. This is accomplished by appropriate exercise routines along with proper nutrition.
7. Cigarette smoking may be a cause for being underweight. The underweight smoker has a poor outlook in terms of longevity.
8. Coffee, tea and caffeine containing colas may have a mild effect in preventing a needed weight gain.
9. Estrogen is important in enabling a woman to develop normal fat pads. But if the estrogen level is normal, taking additional estrogen is not helpful or advisable.

10. Testosterone stimulates muscular development, but the use of testosterone or steroids by normal males is often harmful.
11. If you inherited the genes to be thin, it is probably not a good idea to try to gain weight you are not supposed to carry. It is better to accept your individual characteristics and be content.

Chapter 19

A Look at the Future

Our understanding of how the body balances calories and acts as an energy converter is constantly expanding. As new facts are learned, old methods are outdated and have to be replaced. That doesn't alter the basic laws of nature, but does improve our methods of using them to our advantage. An understanding of the energy balance system suggests what you can expect in the future.

Reprogramming the Computer

It's clear that the brain is in control of your energy balance. All the details of how it does this, and which nerve cells and receptors control which aspect of the complex interaction, are not known. But we do know that brain chemistry has a lot to do with it. This opens the door to finding ways to influence the brain's function in controlling your calorie balance. We already know that certain medicines are associated with body weight gain. It should be recognized that this is done within the laws of energy conservation. The medicines simply stimulate the appetite, so that calorie consumption greatly exceeds calorie use. The weight gain associated with monamine oxidase inhibitors, used to treat depressions, is a good example of what happens. As they allow the levels of noradrenaline to increase in the brain, that stimulates the appetite. Weight gain will follow, unless one maintains strict adherence to a diet that prevents this.

Is there a way to reset the body's thermostat? When the thermostat is set higher, the metabolic turnover of calories of heat is increased. This

251

also stimulates the body to lose calories, and unless calorie intake is increased, that can result in loss of body fat.

The possibilities involved with reprogramming the brain are endless. Whatever is developed must be something that does not interfere with the normal, healthy function of the body's cells. Inducing under-nutrition, and shutting down the normal metabolic system, by whatever means, is not likely to be a step forward in the sensible management of being overweight.

Correcting Inherited Genes

One of the important frontiers of medicine is learning how the genes influence the body. There is ample evidence that genes which you inherit exert a major, if not the dominant, influence on whether you will be fat or thin, and, if they cause you to be fat, where the fat will go. The possibilities of altering the genes exist. It is now possible to insert a different gene into the genetic pool and affect the genetic makeup. Does that mean the day will come when the genes involved in stimulating you to be overweight can be changed? Perhaps. It could also mean that the genes that cause middle-aged spread can be controlled. It may even mean that the genes that control your life script, and hence your life span, may be subject to control. Do not underestimate the possibilities of science.

The genetic factors related to being overweight or underweight are just beginning to be discovered. It is quite likely that there are several different genetic possibilities. There are different genes involved in different strains of obese mice. Some have a combination gene for being diabetic and obese. Others only have genes for being obese. It would be surprising to find that there is only one genetic variation to cause being overweight, when in your life span you will gain weight, and where the fat deposits will go.

Correcting the Disease Genes

We do know that many of our most important diseases are associated with genes. The formation of increased amounts of cholesterol and LDL-cholesterol that lead to fatty-cholesterol blockage of arteries is influenced by genes. So is adult-onset diabetes. Right now, we have only a few ways to help people who have these problems. One of the most effective ways is through body weight control. Keeping a person thin helps keep certain gene combinations from causing the body to produce too much cholesterol or too much LDL-cholesterol. Today, we use low-fat, low-cholesterol diets, exercise, body weight reduction and medicines to help lower, LDL-cholesterol and raise HDL-cholesterol, or to lower blood glucose levels.

These are stop-gap procedures, but they are the best and safest methods we have to do this at present. If we were able to change genes and lower cholesterol, LDL-cholesterol, blood glucose and blood pressure, we would not need to rely on diets, exercise or some of the medicines used to counteract these problems. That probably will happen. Until that day arrives, though, it is essential for people with these problems to follow measures that keep their bodies lean, even if they cause undernutrition, to reverse processes that can be life-threatening.

Eliminating Hot Calories

The most neglected area of controlling overweight has been in how the body eliminates calories. It seems incredible that so much attention has been given to decreasing "calories in" while so little effort has been made regarding how to influence "calories out." Most of the public, and I suspect quite a few professionals, have not even thought about the well established fact that the way the body eliminates calories is almost entirely through losing heat. And most of those calories leave the body through the skin. This is not a matter of professional debate, but a well-established fact.

Fortunately, exercise does stimulate the loss of calories of heat. That is a major factor in the effectiveness of exercise in helping to control body weight. It is true that being exposed to cold will help eliminate calories through your skin. Clothing largely defeats that aspect of eliminating calories. Not many people would want to make themselves cold and uncomfortable to eliminate calories. However, the combination of lowered temperatures, less clothing and increased physical activity has merit.

Are there other ways to stimulate the loss of calories? There must be. We know that medicines used to treat fever will cause a loss of body heat through the skin. That is one of the functions of salicylate, found in ordinary aspirin. The catch is that many of these do not cool the body unless you already have a fever.

Alcohol is well known for its effect in causing a flush and a feeling of being hot. The problem with alcohol is that it also contains enough calories so that its heat-losing effects may be offset by adding calories to the system. Is there an optimal level of alcohol that would produce the increased blood flow through the skin without having other bad effects on the body? This may be a clue as to how new medicines can be developed that would do this without causing harm?

Are there ways to stimulate the brain's basic control over heat loss? Probably. Remember the cat experiment, in which diathermy was used to selectively warm the hypothalamus. The cat began to pant and its paws began to sweat. New agents that affect brain chemistry without unacceptable side effects may be a future advance in controlling weight problems.

New Ways to Increase Metabolism

Once the body has burned foods to carbon dioxide and water, there is no way the heat can safely be retained in the body. It must be eliminated. Are there ways to increase this action, so that you can literally speed up the energy release process by your cells? We know that an excess of thyroid hormone will do this, but it has unwanted and dangerous side-effects when used in sufficient quantity to cause weight loss, including causing a loss of important body protein and heart irregularities. However, it provides a clue. Is it possible to develop related medicines that will speed metabolism a desirable amount without the harmful side-effects?

New Ways to Empty Fat Cells

The discovery that fat cells have different types of receptors, which control the loading and unloading of the cell with fat, offers an intriguing way to eliminate fat deposits. Studies in the laboratory suggest that it may be possible to greatly speed up the emptying of fat-filled cells. At present, those cells with $alpha_2$ receptors are highly resistant to unloading. That is why those "love handles" and heavy thighs persist, in spite of everything you do to get rid of them. Just as there is a suggestion that beta-blocker medicines may prevent the unloading of certain fat cells, there may be other medicines that will stimulate the release of fat.

Developing ways to empty the fat cells may not be enough. Remember that the amount of body fat you have is greatly influenced by the brain. Those empty fat cells may merely stimulate the brain to increase your appetite. The chemical battle that may result between stimulating your fat cells to empty, and the brain's effort to fill them, will probably end with the brain winning. But the removal of fat cells would remove any opportunity they would have to trigger the brain's appetite-stimulation mechanism. In the future, the role of surgery to remove fat cells may have more application than is apparent at the moment. And it may be far superior to the current surgical approaches of bypassing the intestine or the stomach.

Identifying Those at Risk

The fat cell story and the genetic story offer new opportunities for preventive medicine—the prevention of becoming overweight. If both parents are overweight, a child has an 80 percent chance of also being overweight. It seems rather simple to help these children early in life to avoid developing habits that would increase their tendency to be overweight. Some studies suggest that there is an increase in fat cells in children who are overfed during the first two years of life. It may be unwise to allow a child to be fat in those early years. Avoiding this, and preventing the development of an excess number of fat cells, may help to prevent being overweight later in life. The same applies to the period of puberty. This is also believed to be a time when there can be a proliferation of fat cells. While it is important for the child to avoid getting fat at these stages of development, during both stages the child needs an adequate number of calories to support growth. The goal is to prevent overfeeding to the point where body fat cells develop.

Doing fat cell biopsies, and studying the number and characteristics of the cells under a microscope, may help to plot the course of what is happening. In the adult, such studies may also help to define the cause of being overweight, and whether it is from overeating, a lack of physical activity, a genetic condition, or a combination of these factors.

Some Improvements in Lifestyle

Today, it is difficult for most people to know how many calories they are consuming. Food labels are part of the problem. People have a right to know how many calories are in each gram or ounce of their food. They need to know how much is fat, which kind of fat, and how much is protein and carbohydrate. This is vital information for people who need to control their calorie consumption, and the source of the calories. There are too many ways that extra calories can be slipped into prepared foods. Often, people do not know whether they are getting calorie-rich foods or calorie-poor foods. One of the things that can be accomplished, without any great new scientific breakthroughs, is proper food labeling that will include this vital information.

The fitness boom has been a big help in making people healthier—safely eliminating calories and, in most cases, increasing their metabolically-active tissue. There needs to be more information regarding how many calories different forms of exercise really use, and the best ways to use exercise for weight control. What are the tradeoffs between short-duration, intensive activity, compared to long-duration, low-intensity activity, or frequent short periods of moderate activity? The effects in relation to the heart have been rather well studied, but the relation to calorie balance has not been well defined. Part of this is because of failure to measure the long-term effects of activity on metabolism, long after the activity itself is over.

We also need more information on how to improve strength training, and a greater public awareness of its important role in building the amount of metabolically-active tissue in the body. New ways to improve the growth of muscle are important, but this must be done safely, using methods other than taking anabolic steroids or using gimmicks that may be detrimental to one's health.

New Foods

If you think about it, there have been a number of changes in the foods available that are helpful in limiting your calorie intake. A good example is protein fortified skim milk, which actually provides more calcium and more complete protein with less calories than regular milk. It is also a low-fat, low-cholesterol product.

There are already a number of substitutes for sugar and other sweets, though there are mixed reviews on these; they can be used in selected individuals to help curtail excessive calorie intake. Fat is often the main source of excess calories. It contains more calories per weight than any other food. It is everywhere. People like fat, particularly sweet fat as found in candy and ice cream. A large segment of the public behaves like the ordinary laboratory rat that is fed calorie-rich snacks and gains weight. The ideal solution to this problem is to provide fats that do not contain an excess of calories. "Come on now, that is impossible," you are thinking. Not only is it possible, but it has been done. About 20 years ago, Procter & Gamble developed a substance called sucrose polyester. It will eventually be sold under the name of Olestra. Sucrose polyester is an example of what may be possible in the future. It is a very large fat molecule, made by attaching fatty acids to the long carbon chain of ordinary table sugar. This large molecule evidently is not broken down by the digestive system, and is too large to be absorbed into the circulation. The result is that it never gets into the body. If it doesn't get into the body, it cannot provide calories. Such a substance could be used in place of our calorie-rich fats in such foods as ice cream, candy, spreads and fatty salad dressings. It can be used in food preparation anywhere that you could use any of the cooking oils or fats. Imagine, low calorie French fries. The possibilities are endless.

In the 20 years that Procter & Gamble has studied Olestra they have found that it will effectively lower body weight, simply by reducing calorie intake, and it also will lower total cholesterol by about 15 percent.

Developing such products is not easy. One has to be sure they do not interfere with normal absorption of sufficient minerals and vitamins. Olestra will contain some vitamin supplements to adjust for any problems of this sort. It is important that too many of these low-calorie items don't find their way into foodstuffs, or a lot of people would not be getting enough calories to support their energy requirements. Olestra is currently under review by the Food and Drug Administration and may be approved within the next two years.

Still another fat substitute is Simplesse. This product contains no fat. It is made from the protein in egg white and milk. By changing it mechanically into spheres, it provides the feel and taste of fat. It cannot be cooked, but it can be used in such products as ice cream. It is a product of the NutraSweet Company.

A Change in Attitude

One of the most pressing needs in nutrition today is a better understanding of the normal aspects of body weight. There is so much emphasis on appearance that health is often neglected. It is important for many people to stay lean for medical reasons. But it is equally important for people to understand what undernutrition does to them. For many people, it is all right to have a little body fat. It may even be healthier for some people to be a little heavy.

Whether excess body weight is a medical problem or not depends on what is actually happening to *your* own body, not how body weight affects a group of individuals. I like to say we should individualize, not generalize. The public needs to understand that being "overweight" *is* a medical problem when it is associated with high cholesterol levels, high LDL-cholesterol levels, high blood glucose levels and high blood pressure. A perfectly healthy person who is heavy may not need to lose body fat. A word of caution is necessary. One needs to be careful to have optimal medical findings that are associated with the least risk of future disease, rather than just "normal" findings that are associated with a high rate of disease in our affluent society. Just because it is normal to have a heart attack doesn't make it desirable.

Fortunately, we are already beginning to see a renewed recognition that age does have a relation to body weight. No doubt, this is controlled by the brain's biological clock that determines life span and body weight. Unless there are associated medical findings that need attention, it may be all right to gain weight as you reach 60 and beyond. Of course, it is important to keep up the kind of exercise pattern that will help you maintain your muscles, as part of your metabolically-active, fat-free body weight. If you allow your muscles to decrease in size as you get older, that can contribute to being overweight. If a person has medical problems associated with being overweight, just being older doesn't mean he can ignore his overweight condition. But it will be good if older people in good health are able to gain a normal amount of healthy weight as the years go by, and not forced into undernutrition or made to feel guilty about their body weight.

Summary 19

1. A future approach to managing body weight could involve how

the brain controls your calories consumed, your calories used and your quantity of body fat.

2. Influencing inherited genes offers an approach to controlling body weight. That may include correcting faulty genes that cause combined problems of being overweight, along with having diabetes, high blood pressure and perhaps other medical problems.

3. Since one type of fat cells seems to play an important role in causing fat deposits resistant to usual weight control methods, it may be possible to use medicines to stimulate these fat cells to release their fat stores.

4. Ways to identify those at risk of becoming overweight early in life may make it possible to start preventing obesity at an early age.

5. Better food labels are needed in our modern world of prepared foods so people can tell how many calories of what they are eating. That is essential in controlling the number of calories people consume.

6. More knowledge is needed about how to ensure and maintain good muscle development and strength, and to use exercise properly to build a good metabolic furnace that will help maintain energy levels and prevent being overweight.

7. New foods that satisfy the human urge for fats, sweets and starches without overloading calorie consumption are either here or being developed.

8. There is a great need for a better public and individual awareness of what causes some people to have more body fat than others. An appreciation that this is a natural characteristic for some people at various stages of life should help to eliminate the unrealistic and almost universal prejudice and discrimination against "fat" people in our society.

9. People need to understand the dangers of undernutrition in relation to their enjoyment of life and to their health.

Chapter 20

How to Win the Weighting Game

Over 90 percent of people who go on a diet and lose weight regain the weight they have lost. It is always discouraging to be one of those 90 percent, but it is worse to lose weight that you need for good health and become one of the dietary victims of undernutrition. If you are going to play the weighting game, you need to have a clear idea of the best way to do it, while maintaining or improving your health. With the information you have learned in this book, you can do it.

Do You Need to Lose Weight?

Before you even start a weight-loss program, you need to do some hard thinking. The first question you should ask yourself is, "Do I really need to lose weight?" In a surprising number of instances, the answer is no. In arriving at a reasonable answer, you need to think about your family history. It will give you some indication whether your slightly heavy body is meant to be that way or not. For women, it is more common to have a reasonable amount of fat than it is to be skinny. Even if you have a family history of heavyweights, that doesn't mean you can't do something about it, but it does mean you need to be more careful to avoid becoming a victim of undernutrition.

The second question is, "Do I have any medical findings that would be helped if I lost weight?" Perhaps the most important reason for losing excess pounds of body fat is one or more medical findings that indicate the presence of disease, or an increased risk of disease that can be decreased by losing excess fat. That means you need to know

261

your blood total cholesterol, your HDL-cholesterol and your blood glucose levels. You also need to know what your blood pressure is. As this would suggest, a visit to the doctor's office before embarking on a weight-loss program is advisable. There is another reason. If you just want to lose a few pounds, you can do it on your own, following basic principles. But if you really have a lot of body fat to lose, you will need medical supervision. That is even more important if you already have medical problems.

The third question, and the one that usually counts, is, "Will I look better if I lose weight?" Don't kid yourself. If you want to look better, that is fine, but don't allow that to cause you to force yourself into an unhealthy situation with undernutrition. Today's style may mean you would look better if you were lean, but that is more a matter of current concepts of style. It may not improve your appearance to be thin if you lose your spark because you have turned your energy machine down too low. When you have forced yourself to be thin, your body may be "laughing on the outside and crying on the inside." There is a lot of wisdom in the old saying that you can't judge a book by its cover.

Do You Need to Diet?

You now know that there are a lot of different factors that can lead to being overweight. One of those can be eating too much. Try to assess what is causing you to be overweight. Are you hot and overweight? If so, too many calories are likely to be at least part of the cause.

The next stop is to keep a diet diary. List everything you eat and drink, and try to establish what your usual calorie intake is. If you need help, get it. Your diet diary is the single most important clue as to whether you are overweight because of eating too much. If you find that your calorie intake is less than 2,000 calories a day for a woman of average size, or 2,500 calories for a man of average size, the chances are that you are not overeating. The lower your calorie intake, the less likely it is the cause of being overweight.

So, you have decided to limit your calorie intake to help you shed some pounds. How many calories should your diet include? That is where you are apt to get into trouble. A low-calorie diet really shouldn't be less than 1,600 calories a day for most women, or less than 1,800 calories for men. Even that restriction is on the low side, and can cause you to become a victim of undernutrition.

If you have any doubts about what your calorie intake should be, have your near-basal oxygen consumption measured, as previously suggested. Find out what your near-basal calorie requirements really are, instead of guessing. You will be glad you did.

What kind of diet should you follow? You don't need a fad diet. People who use these are usually the ones who end up regaining the weight they have lost. Keep in mind that you want to use a plan that can be the basis for your regular diet after you have reached your weight goal. You can simply add to the basic diet, when your metabolic system has improved to the point that you can use more calories without regaining body fat. As a starting point, you can use the basic diet I have provided for you and add what foods you need to adjust it to the right caloric level for you. When you do that, try to include at least 70 grams of good quality protein a day. Why? Because you are going to need to work on building your active metabolic tissue. That means muscle, and you will need some extra protein for that. Your program will probably increase your muscle weight less than a pound a week, so 70 grams of protein should be adequate. To support a major-muscle-building program with strength exercises, you might need 100 grams of protein a day. That is more than necessary to develop one pound of muscle a week. That amount will provide a safety factor for the biological inefficiency of the process. Gaining a half-pound of muscle a week would be outstanding for most people.

The most important type of foods to eliminate from your diet are fats. Remember that they contain more calories than anything else. Just eliminating all the fats you can will do more to help you develop a good, balanced diet—which can still be satisfying and provide the basis for your permanent diet—than any other thing you can do. You need very little fat to meet the body's small requirements. Fat is not used to build body protein and fatty acids cannot be converted to glucose.

Another overlooked point about dietary fat was demonstrated by the study that showed that some overweight people responded differently to fat. When they consumed fat, it was not converted to heat. That means it was not used. It also means it was readily stored as body fat. But people who were not overweight used fat like all other foods, and burned it to release energy. This is a strong argument for limiting the fat in your diet, especially if you are overweight. If I had to make just one single diet recommendation to people who are overweight and need to reduce, it would be, *GET THE FAT OUT!*

It is worth mentioning again that you should not use alcohol. In my experience, very few people who insisted on one or more daily cocktails were able to lose body fat and keep it off. Alcohol, like fat, provides little other than calories. Actually, it is processed in your metabolic system as if it were a fat, not a sugar. It cannot be used to form either glucose or amino acids for proteins.

You may want to limit the concentrated carbohydrates such as sweets and starches. That does not mean you need to eliminate carbohydrates. Far from it. They may be your most helpful foods. Remember that your brain will need 125 grams of glucose a day, even if you don't use it. If your diet doesn't provide it, your liver will take some of those proteins you need for muscle and convert them to glucose. So be sure to get your 100 grams of good-quality protein, limit your fat and round out the rest of your diet with a variety of carbohydrate foods.

That carbohydrate will help you keep your muscle glycogen up, too, and that will help with your exercise program. Remember that at the onset of exercise, your muscles will use mostly glycogen before starting to use fatty acids. If you don't maintain your levels of muscle glycogen, you are apt to tire easily.

Avoid those diets that restrict your calories excessively, and that can include the popular 1,200 calorie diets. Most of those low-calorie diets are recommended for only a few weeks, anyway. As you have seen, because of the many ways your body has of controlling your calorie balance, it is easy to regain those pounds just as soon as you finish one of those diets. Those overly restrictive diets are a sure way to be one of the 90 percent of the people who lose when playing the weighting game. If you restrict your calories too much, you will lose body protein from your metabolically-active tissue. That means you will have less tissue that uses calories and gives you energy. As a result, you are even more likely to get overweight after one of those very low-calorie diets.

Don't use any of the low-calorie, low-carbohydrate diets. They do not help. They will not create any magic to help you lose any more fat over a several week period than any other diet which contains the same number of calories. You need to remember that you need to make a permanent change in your diet, if it is the cause of your being overweight, and if you want to stay at your new weight level.

Eat breakfast. For years, I wondered why, because there were no hard facts to justify that old admonition. The answer is in what happens to your glycogen stores overnight, while you are not eating. In the morning, your liver will be about 75 percent depleted of glycogen. It will already be using your body protein to manufacture glucose. If you want to protect your body protein, you had better provide some carbohydrate early in the morning to replace that glucose. Your brain will function better too, as it needs that glucose to maintain its ability to do all the complex tasks required of it. If you have a low-carbohydrate breakfast or no-carbohydrate breakfast you may not be doing your brain a favor. Your liver will still have to convert protein to glucose to feed your brain. Fruit and cereal is a good way to start the day.

Try to eliminate the conditioned response. We are a society that runs on a time basis. That makes it difficult to do this, but it is true that if you eat at specific times, you will be hungry at those times. If you can learn to eat only when you are hungry, not just by the clock, you can help tone down that conditioned response to eat.

Do You Need More Physical Activity?

If you do not feel hot, and particularly if you feel cold, you are apt to be overweight because of insufficient physical activity. The reason many people have put on extra pounds of fat they do not need is that they really do not have enough physical activity to use even a modest and healthy intake of food. A good place to start on this problem is to keep an activity diary. List what you do each day in order, then assess how many calories all those activities really require. If you have an office job, or your work requires sitting most of the time, the chances are that your job is not requiring any more energy than if you were simply relaxing around the house. The simple truth is that the energy requirements for many occupations today are less than a person's nonworking, nonsleeping hours. When you are putting together your activity diary, don't forget to include your hours of sleeping. The more hours you sleep, the fewer calories you use. That includes time sleeping in front of the TV.

As a guide to how many calories you are using for your level of activity, you can use 20 calories per hour spent in very light activity such as sitting, standing, sewing, cooking, playing a musical instrument, or work that involves standing or sitting, such as painting or driving. For light work, such as walking at less than three miles an hour, electrical trades, garage work, carpentry, restaurant work or golf, use 110 calories per hour. For moderately heavy activity, including walking 3.5 to 4.0 miles an hour, yard work, scrubbing floors, cycling, skiing, tennis or dancing, you can use 210 calories an hour. If you are doing heavier work than that, for any length of time, you are probably getting enough physical activity, and you probably have no problem with being overweight, unless you are consuming a lot of extra calories.

If you realize that you are not really using many calories from physical activity, you need to develop an exercise program, as I have outlined in chapter 12, Why Exercise Is Essential. You need some endurance exercise, and that can start with walking. Just remember that the endurance exercises will drive your catabolic system and help you eliminate calories. Using them to maintain your proper calorie balance is far more healthy than restricting your calories, but endurance exercises are not the total answer to your exercise needs.

Unless you are doing work that helps you develop good strong muscles, you do need an exercise program to develop and maintain your muscle size and strength. Yes, this does include women. Perhaps I should say it especially includes women, because so many women do not have a lifestyle that requires them to use strength. As a result, they are especially likely to have small, underdeveloped muscles. A good calisthenic program, using the body weight for resistance, is helpful in this regard. It is not necessary to be as well-developed as Arnold Schwarzenegger, but the more healthy muscle tissue you have, the greater your near-basal calorie utilization will be, and the less likely you will be to develop fat deposits. The failure to include any strength type activity in your exercise program is a big mistake when you are planning your lifestyle to avoid excess body fat.

One Last Thought

If you follow these relatively simple rules, *you can win the weighting game* and maintain your proper, healthy weight for life. My last recommendation is that while you are playing the game, and regardless of what anyone tells you,

DON'T FIGHT YOUR BODY!